Living a Longer Healthier Life

The companion guide to
Dr. A's Habits of Health

Living a Longer
Healthier Life

The companion guide to
Dr. A's Habits of Health

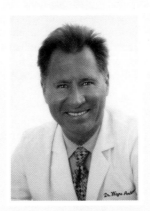

Dr. Wayne Scott Andersen

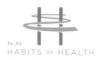

Dr. A's
HABITS of HEALTH

P.O. Box 3301
Annapolis, Maryland 21403
www.drwayneandersen.com

First Edition
Printed in the United States of America

30 29

ISBN: 978-0-9819146-2-6 paperback

Design by Dede Cummings Design
Production by Carolyn Kasper
DCDESIGN / BRATTLEBORO, VERMONT

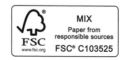

MIX
Paper from
responsible sources
FSC® C103525

Printed on Paperfect paper with pulp that comes from FSC (Forest Stewardship Council) certified forests, managed forests that guarantee responsible environmental, social, and economic practices. Made with a chlorine-free process (ECF: Elemental Chlorine Free).

To those who are thinking of taking the journey . . . join us!

To those who are on the path . . . welcome!

To those who have created optimal health . . . lead!

Creating health for ourselves and our loved ones—and then reaching out and helping others—is a powerful grassroots approach to healing an un- healthy world. I am in awe of the ever-growing number of coaches and health care professionals who are leading the way to a healthier, longer life for so many. Thank you!

We have only just begun to create . . .

CONTENTS

Section Two The Habits of Reaching and Maintaining a Healthy Weight   55

Section Three The Habits of Optimal Health and Longevity   111

CONTENTS

INTRODUCTION

This workbook serves as the companion guide to *Dr. A's Habits of Health,* a comprehensive manual designed to give you control of your daily habits and behaviors in order to create a life of vibrancy and optimal health. The main text will be referenced often in this guide.

But you will find much more here than simple exercises and activities. *Living a Longer, Healthier Life* is actually a critical piece of self-actualization. It's the difference between just reading about creating health and actually doing it. In fact, "just do it" is our whole approach.

Habits of Health—those daily habits that create and support optimal health—can only be developed through repetition. Together, we'll explore different ways to make that happen. Some techniques will resonate with you and become your favorites, and others may not. That's okay.

One of the methods I have found to be extremely helpful is the powerful dynamic of structural tension. These techniques are derived from the work of my friend and mentor Robert Fritz, a master in the creative process. I have adopted this work with his permission and have successfully helped thousands of people create health in their lives.

The choices that form the foundation of optimal health are different for each of us. What we do have in common is that we must each take individual responsibility for our health. Big business, government, even the traditional medical community have failed to deliver on their promises of healthier living, despite today's surplus of technology and advanced medications.

That's why we've designed *Dr. A's Habits of Health* and this companion guide as roadmaps to help you find your way to better health and take back the life you deserve. In them, you'll learn and practice behaviors that will set you on your way to…

LIVING A LONGER, HEALTHIER LIFE

As you prepare for your journey to optimal health, you'll need to:

- Recognize the influence of your environment on your current health
- Create a new microenvironment that supports better health
- Understand the power of habits in all aspects of your life
- Determine to take responsibility for your health
- Make the fundamental choice to create optimal health in your life
- Learn my system for implementing these new behaviors into your life

HOW TO USE THIS COMPANION GUIDE

The trouble with the world is not that people
know too little, but that they know so many things
that ain't so.

—MARK TWAIN

This guide is structured to serve as the basis for a lifetime of learning about and practicing health—sort of like a primer.

When you paint a surface, you first need to prepare it with a coat of primer. Slopping paint onto a chipped or weathered surface is a recipe for a poor outcome. To help you avoid falling into the trap that Mark Twain observes above, I've created a series of progressive lessons for your health journey. Section one is designed to make sure you're grounded in knowing where you are right now, where you're going, and how to get there. Then, in sections two and three, you'll learn the essential Habits of Health in a logical order that will take you to your healthy weight, to optimal health, and beyond.

To make sure these healthy habits become a lasting part of your life, you'll learn them through a formula I call the *cycle of success*. This cycle starts by developing a clear understanding of the principles behind each lesson by reading corresponding chapters from *Dr. A's Habits of Health*, which I've listed at the beginning of each chapter. You'll then learn a series of exercises, skills, and daily choices that will help you engrain the Habits of Health.

Then you'll start the process all over again!

Learn — Do — Review — Correct — Repeat

This is the cycle of success. Each time you complete this cycle, you're reinforcing the Habits of Health and instilling continuous improvement—a process called *kaizen* in Japan, where it was applied to the auto industry with huge success.

In other words, your goal is not just to complete a lesson and say, "I'm finished," but to repeat these lessons, making small adjustments to your actions and choices. As you improve and celebrate your successes, you gain the momentum that will help propel you toward optimal health—and serve as a powerful method of self-improvement that will give you the tools to adapt to a rapidly changing world.

Before we get started, I want to share with you another valuable method that can help you process these lessons and accelerate your success. It's called *learning through modeling*. Your model may be a coach, a mentor, or someone else who's already living the Habits of Health. By teaming up with someone who's well along the path to optimal health, you don't need to go it alone and you can learn from their mastery.

So let's put the wheels in motion!

How do you eat an elephant?
One bite at a time!

I know that starting something new can create anxiety. But don't worry—I have you covered.

This Companion Guide is divided into three sections:

Section One

The first seven lessons are designed to prepare you to make a permanent shift in your health. They'll help you hone your axe so you have the knowledge and skills to succeed in what you (and so many others) have failed in the past—reach a healthy weight and give yourself radiant optimal health. We're going to make sure we equip you with all the tools to incorporate the Habits of Health into your life.

The lessons on habits contain brand new, essential material to help move you forward from thought into action. We'll then return to the health assessment from *Dr. A's Habits of Health* to reinforce your understanding of how your current habits are affecting your health. You'll then build skills to help you decide what you want, develop the proper motivation, and gain the tools you need to guide your choices, as well as the discipline to make optimal health a reality. Finally, we'll outline the major foundational pieces that pave the way to a healthier, longer life.

Section Two

The second seven lessons follow directly along with corresponding chapters in *Dr. A's Habits of Health*. In them, you'll learn how to use the techniques you learned in the first section to bring each Habit to Health alive for you. You'll begin by adding the Habits of Health that focus on comprehensive weight control.

Section Three

The final seven lessons will help take you to optimal health and, if you like, help you implement an advanced plan to potentially help you live longer.

Throughout the Companion Guide, you'll find a number of page references from the main text. You can use these references to help you locate the answers to the questions in this workbook. **Note that the abbreviation HOH refers to the main text, *Dr. A's Habits of Health*.**

For those of you who learn visually Dr. A's HOH Video Series can provide an opportunity to learn directly from Dr. Andersen. He will take you through the series of lessons, and provide a coach and client interaction to help you incorporate the Habits of Health into your life.

Optimal health can become a reality. The Habits of Health are standing by, ready to bring radiant health into your life. Today's the best possible day to start.

Just do it!

IMPORTANT

Before you begin, I recommend that you schedule a visit to see your primary care provider. In Appendix A, you'll find a sheet of information to give your physician that explains this "health makeover" you're doing. It's also available for download at www.habitsofhealth.net.

Section One
The Tools to Create
a Healthy New Life

LESSON 1 ▸ Your Changing World

Leave behind the world of obesity for one of vibrant, long-lasting health

BEFORE YOU BEGIN
Read Chapters 1 and 2 in *Dr. A's Habits of Health*

GOALS
- Understand how our innate design conflicts with our world
- Learn which factors cause us to accumulate fat
- Identify a new path to create health vs. react to disease

Our body's innate design has served us well—for our first 3 million or so years on earth. Our elaborate system of energy conservation and 40 billion fat cells helped us use every calorie efficiently, and hoard energy when needed.

We searched and hunted all day for our food, most of which was energy sparse, meaning that it delivered a moderate amount of calories accompanied by a large amount of healthy noncaloric material such as water and fiber. Once in a while we were fortunate to find a form of food that was energy dense, such as a large animal, and we and our clan would eat and eat until our bellies were full. Those extra fat cells gobbled up and stored all that excess energy for the future, when times were lean.

Usually, back then, our daily calorie consumption matched the effort we expended to get those calories, enabling us to maintain a balance of energy in and energy out. We may not have lived long, but we were lean, mean, fighting machines right until the day we fell off a cliff, stepped on a poisonous insect, or became lunch for a saber-toothed tiger.

OUR ENERGY BALANCE 10,000 YEARS AGO

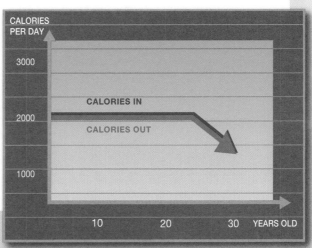

3

Fast-forward to today, and things are altogether different. Modern food technology has made energy-dense food cheap, abundant, and great tasting. Add to that a never-ending stream of energy-saving devices, and our energy management system just can't get the job done anymore.

Just look at the increasing gap between calories in and calorie out in our modern world:

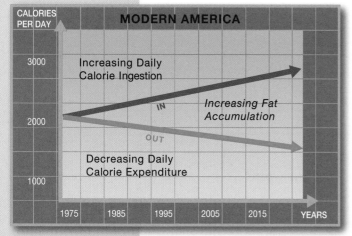

OUR ENERGY BALANCE TODAY

So while our natural tendency is to store energy, our bodies haven't adapted to living in a world with constant exposure to abundant calories. And because our bodies are designed to conserve energy, we gravitate to machines and devices that rob us of the muscle-building movement that could help offset that higher intake.

Let's see how this applies to your life.

COMPARE YOUR DAILY FOOD CHOICES WITH YOUR DAILY ACTIVITIES DURING THE COURSE OF ONE DAY.

FOOD AND DRINK INGESTED	ENERGY EXPENDED (e.g., exercise, sports)
(calories in during one day)	(calories out during one day)

If you're like most people today, your "calories in" space filled up a lot quicker than your "calories out"—and if you actually measured your totals, your energy intake would exceed your energy expenditure.

Add to this imbalance the fact that we lose on average a pound of muscle per year after age twenty. Since each pound consumes 50–70 calories of energy in a twenty-four hour period, by the time we're forty we've lost about 1,400 calories of energy expenditure a day! Although this rate will slow as we age and continue to lose muscle mass, its negative effect on our energy balance and health will continue. And because modern medicine has eliminated many infectious diseases, our life span has been extended significantly—so as we grow older and become more sedentary, our bodies are carrying an unhealthy amount of fat.

YOUR JOURNEY TO SARCOPENIA, or "Honey, I've Shrunk My Muscles!"

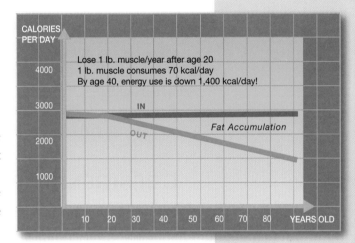

If you're over 20 and are not on a weight-resistance program or working a labor-intense job, it's a good bet that you're accumulating fat.

On top of which, we're swimming in a sea of what I like to call *nutritional pollution*. Over 90 percent of the food we eat is processed, meaning that in addition to all those energy-dense extra calories, we're eating a diet that's:

1. High glycemic (e.g., high-fructose corn syrup)
2. High fat
3. High in salt
4. High in chemicals

Tomorrow, take note of everything in your diet that comes from processed food.

EXERCISE

Read the ingredients of everything you put in your body tomorrow. Beginning at zero, tabulate your score as follows: If the label doesn't list one of the four components listed above in the first four ingredients, add 1 to your score. If one of the four components is listed as one of the first four ingredients, subtract 1 from your score.

10 and above	Excellent
6 to 9	Good
1 to 5	Fair
0 to -5	Bad
-5 to -9	Very bad
-10 and below	Inflammatory nightmare

Nutritionally polluted foods raise havoc with our bodies in many ways. Besides providing way too many calories, their high-glycemic content turns on insulin and puts you in a constant fat-storage mode. Along with fat creep, it's a recipe for *metabolic syndrome*—a cluster of symptoms that affects over 70 million people in the U.S. alone. As our body's defenses are overcome, we begin the downward spiral of medication, doctor visits, and hospitalization, all as a result of nutritional pollution and a sedentary lifestyle!

It's probably clear to you by now that if you don't take an active role in making daily choices that support health, you'll soon be on the slippery slope from optimal health to non-sickness to sickness. Technology creates more health-robbing foods and machines, pharmaceutical companies sell sickness, and even the medical community is geared toward reacting to disease once it occurs, not preventing it in the first place. That's why *you* need to take control by taking a path that leads you away from our obesigenic world and toward health. And that's just the path you're starting on now!

Our simple-to-follow plan begins by getting you to a healthy weight. Soon you'll feel better, could possibly reduce certain weight-related medications, and you'll be ready to learn all the Habits of Health.

First, let's take a quick look at your current habits to see where you are right now. (We'll do a more thorough evaluation in lesson 4.)

OBESIGENIC VS. LEPTOGENIC

You may not give much thought to your daily activities and the choices you make. But by becoming aware of *obesigenic* choices (things that make you obese) and *leptogenic* choices (things that make you thin), you can begin to bring health and control into your life.

Below are common obesigenic and leptogenic situations and choices. Put a star next to the good choices, and an X next to the poor choices that lead to disease.

A plus sign (+) indicates a Habit of Health. A minus sign (-) indicates a Habit of Disease.

_____Eating a substantial breakfast every morning (+)

_____Having three meals a day (-)

_____Using the stairs when possible (+)

_____Having only coffee or orange juice for breakfast (-)

_____Parking far away from the store and walking (+)

_____Watching TV after 10:00 p.m. nightly (-)

_____Taking a short power nap (5 minutes) when tired (+)

_____Taking a nap in the afternoon (-)

_____Exercising 5–7 days weekly (+)

_____Eating more pasta and rice (-)

_____Enjoying eating out at least 4–5 times weekly (-)

_____Choosing a salad with chicken instead of a hamburger (+)

_____Getting 4 hours of sleep (-)

_____Getting 7–8 hours of sleep (+)

_____Eating fish at least 2–3 times a week (+)

_____Finishing your meal with dessert (-)

_____Eating more fruits and vegetables (+)

_____Drinking more caffeinated drinks (-)

_____Drinking more diet soda than water (-)

_____Keeping a journal (+)

_____Drinking at least 8 glasses of water per day (+)

_____Choosing healthy-minded friends (+)

_____Eating lots of protein in the form of meat (+)

_____Having a midday candy bar to get you though till dinner (-)

_____Wearing a pedometer daily and tracking your steps (+)

_____Monitoring your weight weekly (+)

_____Planning ahead for your body's daily fuel (+)

_____Wearing clothes with elastic waistbands (-)

_____Choosing potato chips for a snack (-)

_____Eating 5–6 small, low-fat meals daily (+)

How many healthy choices are you currently making?

I'll bet this exercise was pretty easy to complete. You already know the actions that lead to optimal health. Now the real test is . . . are you ready to implement them into your life and change for the better?

WHAT NEW HEALTHY HABITS DO YOU INTEND TO ADOPT AS YOU WORK TOWARD YOUR GOAL OF OPTIMAL HEALTH?

_____

_____

_____

_____

_____

_____

_____

_____

_____

WHAT UNHEALTHY HABITS DO YOU WANT TO LEAVE BEHIND?

_____

_____

_____

_____

_____

_____

_____

_____

_____

_____

_____

_____

_____

Now let's learn more about some of those habits and how they control our lives.

LESSON 2 ▶ The Power of Habits

Adopt new Habits of Health to build a lifetime of vitality

BEFORE YOU BEGIN

The next two lessons have no reading assignments. They are designed to prepare you to implement the lessons that follow into your daily life.

> ### GOALS
> - Understand how habits are formed
> - Learn how to control old habits
> - Find out how to create new habits

We've all tried to break a bad habit, with varying degrees of success. The tenaciousness with which we hold on to behaviors depends on the thickness of the "cable" we have woven, and the strength of our desire to change.

Bad habits can be difficult to break, but fortunately the same is true for good habits!

In this workbook, we focus on creating new healthy habits rather than wasting a energy trying to get rid of the things you don't want. You'll find that over time your old habits, which are no longer serving you, will lose their power.

HOW HABITS ARE FORMED

So, just how do these repeated behaviors come about? And why do they seem to put us on automatic pilot the moment we get up in the morning and as we go to bed leave us wondering. . . . *what happened to the day?*

Habits are repeated behaviors that tend to occur subconsciously. Like so many of our tendencies, they're an important part of our neurological programming that almost always served us well 10,000 years ago. Avoiding meandering off the trail in a forest overrun with poisonous prickly bushes was an important adaptive mechanism that our ancestors learned quickly.

Today, as you're driving home from work, you use a similar engrained habit to guide your car along the safest, quickest route without thinking much about it. Just think how many times you've gotten to your destination lost in thought or a phone

> Habit is a cable; we weave a thread of it every day, and at last we cannot break it.
> — HORACE MANN

conversation and realized that the car practically drove itself. But there was a time years ago, when you were learning to drive, when you were focused and probably a little nervous to perform this now automatic behavior.

Repetition is the key to automating the endless array of routines and habits that dominate our life. In fact, performing an action over and over again actually causes the neurons in our brain to create the programmed pathways that enable us to automate most of our behaviors. It's a simple conditioning system that causes us to perform certain actions when we're given a stimulus or trigger, until those actions becomes automated.

Habits are vital. They prevent us from becoming overwhelmed by the stress of continuous decision making. They help us navigate our lives. We develop a sense of comfort in our routines. And as long as our habits support our health and vitality, they're wonderful servants.

Unfortunately, many of our habits are no longer serving our best interests. Many have developed as a result of our 10,000-year-old design. As we learned in lesson 1, our biological tendencies to store and conserve energy cause us to gravitate toward opportunities to eat and rest. On top of which, our brain's natural response to stress or negative emotions is to seek comfort.

As we go through our day, we are responding to both external and internal triggers that cause us to behave in a certain way. How we respond to these triggers is a complex tapestry of previous conditioning, based on our life experiences. Our job is to recognize the triggers that reinforce habits that don't serve you well, and to replace those habits with ones that guide you to your goal . . . the Habits of Health!

In this companion guide, you'll apply the knowledge you're learning in *Dr. A's Habits of Health* by actually implementing these new habits into your life. We'll do this by equipping you with the most important tool for creating new sustainable, healthy habits—the power of choice.

YOUR DAILY CHOICES

When did you last sit down and evaluate whether your daily choices were bringing you the results you want most? Or has your life become an automatic reaction to whatever's right in front of you? We're going to help you gain control by organizing your life around what matters most to you.

Let's start by doing something you may not have done for a long while—dreaming. If I could wave my wand and give you instant optimal health, with abundant energy and vitality, what would you do?

> Good habits, once established, are just as hard to break as bad habits.
>
> — ROBERT PULLER

LIST FIVE LIFESTYLE EVENTS YOU WOULD REALLY LOVE TO DO. (recreational, travel, entertainment, or family activities that are currently difficult for you, such as playing catch with your children, going whitewater rafting, or climbing to the top of the Statue of Liberty)

1. _____

2. _____

3. _____

4. _____

5. _____

I hope you start visualizing how wonderful life can be once you reach optimal health. (And of course, you don't have to stop at five!) But are the habits you have now likely to get you there?

DO YOUR CURRENT BEHAVIORS SUPPORT OR PREVENT YOUR ABILITY TO FULFILL YOUR DREAMS?

LIFESTYLE EVENT	CURRENT HABITS	
	Supports	Prevents
e.g., play catch		No activity, get short of breath
1.		
2.		
3.		
4.		
5.		

Like many of us, your daily habits may be affecting your health in negative ways. You may not be able to participate in or fully enjoy activities that would bring you joy. And, like many of us, you may as a result seek instant gratification through food, alcohol, TV, and other short-term pleasures.

But over the years, habits like these start to dominate our behaviors, until they become thick cables that are difficult to break. I call these the Habits of Disease. Soon the daily choices that once brought you pleasure start wearing at the very fabric of your life, sapping your energy and vitality.

WHAT SORTS OF HABITS DO YOU RELY ON WHEN YOU'RE UPSET, STRESSED, DEPRESSED, ANGRY, SAD, BORED, TIRED, OR OVERWORKED?

1.
2.
3.
4.
5.

> Habit is either the best of servants or the worst of masters.
>
> — NATHANIEL EMMONS

These actions are comforting strategies. If they support health, your path to your goal may be quite straightforward. But if you regularly comfort yourself with choices that are harmful, it's important to recognize the relationship between those choices and the effect they have on your health.

As a critical care physician, I've stood at the bedside of many people facing death. Believe me, at those moments no one is thinking about the size of their portfolio or what kind of car they drive. Life is a journey that's hard to enjoy without health. To sacrifice our health for a life-style that makes us overworked and overstressed just doesn't make sense.

So I ask you now, and I'll ask you again:

IF YOU HAD A CHOICE TO LIVE IN OPTIMAL HEALTH, WOULD YOU TAKE IT?

ANSWER _____

If the answer is yes, and if you're willing to adopt the Habits of Health, I guarantee that over the next twelve months you'll be healthier, more active, sleep better, eat better... and you just might be happier!

CHANGING YOUR HABITS

So how are you going to change those habits that you've been unable to change in the past? By understanding that these actions aren't *you,* but rather the result of conditioning that began with routines you developed as a child. Your parents, your environment, and your experiences together created your responses to certain stimuli, and those responses in turn created pathways in your brain much like tracks on a dirt road. The more intense the stimulus, the deeper the track. And as you repeated these actions over and over again, they formed deep ruts that your brain continues to follow subconsciously every time a trigger initiates the sequence.

It looks something like this:

Stimulus ⟶ *Action*

Saber-toothed tiger ⟶ *Run*

It doesn't take many intense experiences like these to engrain a response.

Repetition can also create deeply rooted habits that are hard to change:

Watching TV ⟶ *Hungry* ⟶ *Bowl of popcorn*

And soon enough:

Watching TV ⟶ *Bowl of popcorn*

You may have just finished dinner when you sit down to watch TV with a bowl of popcorn, but the stimulus of hunger is no longer necessary. A Habit of Disease has been born.

WHAT AUTOMATIC ROUTINES OR HABITS CAUSE YOU TO GRAZE MINDLESSLY EVEN WHEN YOU'RE NOT HUNGRY?

1. _____
2. _____
3. _____

But remember, many of the actions we've engrained in our brains—riding a bike, for example, or driving—are helpful. And we're now going to engrain a whole new series of Habits of Health!

Let's look at exactly how we're going to help you change your conditioning and lay down a new set of healthy tracks.

1. Identify the foundational choices that support optimal health and implement a plan to incorporate them into your daily choices.

You're already making some daily choices that support your health. You may have learned these by reading, listening, and gathering information as you tried to get healthy in the past.

LIST TEN DAILY CHOICES THAT SUPPORT YOUR HEALTH RIGHT NOW.

1. _____
2. _____
3. _____
4. _____
5. _____
6. _____
7. _____
8. _____
9. _____
10. _____

We're going to help you engrain these healthy choices—and add new ones. Soon your body will regain its balance and you'll be on the road to long-lasting health.

2. Become aware of the daily choices you make that don't support health.

There's no need to blame yourself for these negative habits. You may not have even been aware that certain choices you were making weren't healthy ones. And for those habits that are deeply engrained, we'll explore what stimuli cause them to occur so that you can avoid those conditions or at least minimize their effect.

3. Think long term.

We're an instant gratification society that seeks the immediate pleasure, comfort, or relief that comes from many Habits of Disease. Instead, we're going to teach you how to make choices that support long-term health

4. Create a microenvironment of health.

By removing as many negative stimuli as possible, we'll decrease those triggers that initiate Habits of Disease.

The next lesson will show you how!

LESSON 3 ▶ Harnessing the Habits of Disease

Tame unhealthy behaviors that no longer serve your best interests while you build Habits of Health

BEFORE YOU BEGIN

There is no reading assignment for this lesson. Enjoy it! It's really going to help you tame those unhealthy habits.

> ### GOALS
> - Learn how to break negative behavioral chains
> - Identify bad habits and their triggers
> - Discover a critical tool for stopping negative behaviors in their tracks

My approach is to help people bring radiant health into their lives by creating health, rather than just reacting to disease. So while breaking bad habits isn't our focus, we do want to minimize their effect for now. Over time, the Habits of Health will begin to crowd out those unhealthy behaviors that aren't serving you.

You probably have a pretty good idea of what some of those behaviors are. You may have struggled with them for years, or even decades, trying to break them, failing, getting depressed, and giving it another go.

Let me give you a tip. Have you ever noticed that it's easier to manage bad habits when we're on vacation? You might have even made a whole bunch of resolutions: "When I get home I'm going to. . . ." Why? Because you're away from the triggers that initiate those behaviors—the stressful job, the brutal schedule, the lack of sleep.

No, I can't give you a permanent vacation, but I can help you identify and eliminate those triggers.

BREAKING THE BEHAVIORAL CHAIN

If you've ever reacted to a bad day by eating a whole bag of chips or an entire pint of ice cream, you're not alone. But if you analyze your behavior, you'll discover that eating in this way usually isn't caused by one single event, but rather by a chain of events, known as a *behavioral chain*.

15

Let's say, for example, that you ate a whole bag of cookies one afternoon. On the surface, you simply went to the kitchen, got out the cookies, and started eating. But on closer examination, you can see that a whole series of antecedents led up to this behavior . . . starting, innocently enough, with the clipping of a coupon:

- Clipped a coupon for fifty cents off your favorite cookies.
- Looked through the coupon box while making a shopping list and decided to use the cookie coupon.
- Bought the bag of cookies.
- Put the cookies in the cupboard.
- Had nothing to do on Sunday.
- Felt bored.
- Developed the urge to eat.
- Went to the cupboard and saw the cookies.
- Brought them out, opened them, and ate two while standing at the counter.
- Took the bag into the living room and continued to eat while reading the Sunday paper.
- Finished the whole bag in fifteen minutes.

The good thing about a behavioral chain is that it can be broken at any one of those links, often in several ways. Here are a few:

LINKS OF THE CHAIN	WAYS TO BREAK THE CHAIN
Clipped coupon.	Don't clip any coupon you don't want. (for high-calorie foods, for example!)
Looked through coupon box.	Only look for coupons that match your program foods.
Bought cookies.	Shop from a list. Don't buy cookies!
Placed cookies in front of cupboard.	"Hide" cookies in cupboard or give them to your neighbor.
Nothing to do on Sunday	Plan weekend activities. . . bike, walk, go shopping.
Felt bored.	Have a list of things to get accomplished around the house.
Developed urge to eat.	Wait 15 minutes, drink a big glass of water, have a healthy snack.
Went to kitchen cupboard.	Take a walk. Get out of the house.
Ate out of the bag.	Take out one cookie and put it on a plate. Put bag away. Sit down to eat slowly.

Ate in living room while reading.	Eat only when sitting at the table. Don't get distracted by TV or a book.
Finished cookies in 15 minutes	Slow down and be aware of what you're doing and eating.

Buried in this example are some techniques that can help you keep those unhealthy habits at bay while you learn the Habits of Health.

1. **Identify unhealthy habits.** If you're not conscious of an unhealthy behavior, it will continue.

LIST TEN DAILY CHOICES THAT DON'T SUPPORT YOUR HEALTH, ESPECIALLY THOSE THAT ARE AUTOMATIC.

_____   _____

_____   _____

_____   _____

_____   _____

_____   _____

---

2. **Locate your triggers.** Figure out what internal or external feelings or circumstances initiate unhealthy choices.

LIST EACH UNHEALTHY HABIT SEPARATELY ALONG WITH ITS TRIGGERS.

Habit of Disease   eating ice cream every night

Triggers   watching favorite nightly TV show

Habit of Disease   eating candy at desk

Triggers   boss yelling at me

Habit of Disease #1   _____

Triggers   _____

Habit of Disease #2 _____

    Triggers _____

Habit of Disease #3 _____

    Triggers _____

Habit of Disease #4 _____

    Triggers _____

Habit of Disease #5 _____

    Triggers _____

Habit of Disease #6 _____

    Triggers _____

Habit of Disease #7 _____

    Triggers _____

Habit of Disease #8 _____

    Triggers _____

Habit of Disease #9 _____

    Triggers _____

Habit of Disease #10 _____

    Triggers _____

This will help you minimize the effect of unhealthy behaviors while we work on replacing them with Habits of Health. Let's look at some more ways to control those unhealthy habits.

MORE WAYS TO HARNESS YOUR HABITS

1. Stop——Challenge——Choose

This is one of the most powerful techniques I've found for uncoupling undesirable reactions to events. Use this anytime you become aware of an unhealthy thought, feeling, or action to awaken your conscious thought process and stop your conditioned response in its tracks.

Let's say you're about to eat a whole tray of appetizers at a party because you're nervous. First, *stop*, and take a deep, slow breath to help bring your emotions under control. *Challenge* yourself by thinking about why you're feeling or acting the way you are. Then *choose* the behavior that supports what you really want.

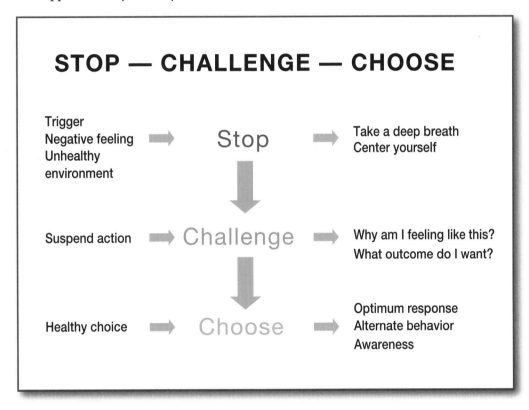

By moving from mindless reaction to conscious awareness, you can avoid actions and behaviors that sabotage your long-term goals.

2. Make time your ally.

Time can be a powerful ally as you build optimal health. As you'll see in the following chart, your daily choices can, over time, lead you from non-sickness to disease. But conversely, time can serve as your ally as you make choices that lead to optimal health.

THE EFFECT OF YOUR CHOICES OVER TIME

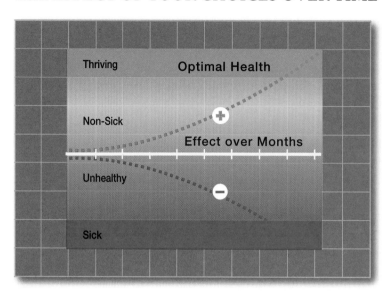

3. Avoid peer pressure and toxic environments.

Do your friends and family follow the same Habits of Disease that you do? Are you hanging out in an unhealthy environment? You'll learn more about modeling later in this workbook, but for now it's a good idea to avoid, as much as possible, any activities, friends, and environments that are conducive to unhealthy behaviors.

4. Keep a journal.

Every time you engage in an activity or make a choice that doesn't support health, write it down. Make note of what triggered the behavior and kept you from controlling the unhealthy choice.

5. Exchange a negative for a positive choice.

Once you've mastered Stop-Challenge-Choose, this technique can help lead you to healthy alternatives. For example, say you're tired at work in the afternoon. You probably habitually grab a cup of coffee, but as you'll learn in the chapter on sleep, this choice can actually exacerbate your lack of energy by robbing you of sleep that night. Instead, recharge naturally by taking a brisk ten-minute walk or resting for five minutes with your eyes closed while listening to relaxing music.

6. Avoid giving the bad habit your energy or focus.

The best way to avoid acting in a certain way is to direct your focus elsewhere.
    Try this quick exercise:

    Look down at the floor!
    Now look up at the ceiling!
    Now, while looking up at the ceiling, can you see the floor?

LIST YOUR PRIMARY CHOICES FOR OPTIMAL HEALTH.

1. _____
2. _____
3. _____
4. _____
5. _____
6. _____
7. _____
8. _____
9. _____
10. _____

CREATING A STRUCTURAL TENSION CHART

We're now going to create a structural tension chart for each of these foundational primary choices as a powerful tool and dynamic motivator for creating optimal health. (For help getting started, review the sample charts in Chapter 4 of *Dr. A's Habits of Health.*)

First, write down what it is you want to bring into reality at the top of the chart. This can be your vision, goal, habit, or primary choice in any aspect of your life. Here, we're focused primarily on the components that will form the foundation for developing a healthier life.

Next, at the bottom of the chart, describe where you are currently in relation to that vision or goal. Draw an arrow from this current reality to your goal, vision, or primary choice. Holding these two conditions in your mind at the same time creates a discrepancy that seeks resolution. This generates a strong desire in you to take action—one that will actually gain momentum as you progress toward your goal and will spur you to learn the secondary choices, or action steps, that will help you reach that goal.

List these secondary choices on the left side of your chart and create a timeline for reaching your goal on the right side. This timeline can be as detailed as you want, or as simple as a target date.

You can even create a structural tension chart for each secondary choice to refine your goals even further and break your progress into baby steps. For example, using the secondary choices in the chart on the next page, you could make eating every three hours your desired goal and your current eating pattern (eating only twice a day) your current reality. In this case, your action steps could include going to the store, making out a schedule, getting some ziplock bags, or ordering meal replacements.

You now have a powerful tool that we'll use in each lesson to help take the Habits of Health from your thoughts to your daily life.

THE FOUNDATION OF A HEALTHY WEIGHT AND NORMAL WAIST SIZE
(Primary Choice)

Healthy Weight

Weight:
BMI:
Waist Circumference:

Secondary Choices

1. Eating every three hours

2. _____

3. _____

4. _____

5. _____

6. _____

7. _____

8. _____

9. _____

90 days

60 days

30 days

Current Reality

Weight:
BMI:
Waist Circumference:

Remember to be specific. Along with reaching a healthy weight, you need to think about reaching a healthy BMI and waist circumference. You can refer back to the health assessment in Chpater 5 of *Dr. A's Habits of Health* for more specific information on these parameters.

While you may not reach your goal in three months, using a timeline allows you track your progress. As you move forward, check your progress regularly. If you're not on track, review your daily choices to make sure they're supporting your primary choice or goal.

EXERCISE

Make a structural tension chart for each of your foundational (primary) choices from the previous exercise.*

---

* All of the following lessons contain a structural tension chart to fill in for each related goal. You can also download copies of this template from www.habitsofhealth.net.

FOUNDATION OF HEALTH _____
   (Primary Choice)

Primary Choice:
_____
_____

Secondary Choices   Timeline

1. _____   _____
2. _____   _____
3. _____   _____
4. _____   _____
5. _____   _____
6. _____   _____
7. _____   _____
8. _____
9. _____
_____
_____

Current Reality

IDENTIFYING YOUR SECONDARY CHOICES

Your secondary choices—exercising daily, for example, or eating proper portions—are the ways you reach your primary goals. See page 33 in *Dr. A's Habits of Health* to review how to write your secondary goals and add these to the left side of your structural tension chart.

Adding a timeline will help keep you on track by creating a sense of urgency. The following sample timeline gives a few examples of ways to move forward.

SAMPLE TIMELINE OF SUCCESS
(choose a date)

Start _____

Get house in order _____

Have healthy foods available _____

Eat every three hours _____

Practice portion control _____

Drink ten glasses of water daily _____

Begin a walking routine _____

Read nightly _____

Sleep eight hours nightly _____

Begin an exercise/motion routine _____

Reach your goal weight _____

Adopt the BeSlim™ philosophy _____

Do something I haven't done in years (bike, play tennis, travel)

_____

Now create your own timeline.

YOUR TIMELINE OF SUCCESS

Start _____ **date**

_____ **by date** _____

_____ **by date** _____

_____ **by date** _____

_____ **by date** _____

_____ **by date** _____

_____ **by date** _____

_____ **by date** _____

_____ **by date** _____

_____ **by date** _____

Goal _____ **by date** _____

FREEING YOUR SELF FROM YOURSELF

As you start on your journey toward a healthy weight, it's important to quiet the "self-talk" that can sabotage your progress—you know, that constant chatter in your head telling you how you're doing, who you should be, what you should do.

With self-talk, you create your own reality, often a false one. If you constantly tell yourself you'll never lose weight, chances are you won't. In fact, you may not even know what you're subconsciously programming into your brain until your actions prove it.

Instead, try to focus on your daily activities, actions, and choices—on the things you want to bring into your life. Focusing on the things you want to create helps you move toward your goals.

EXERCISE

Visualize and write down how you'll feel when you're at your healthy weight and living the Habits of Health. Picture where you want to be three months from now . . . maybe riding a bike with your children, dressed in shorts and a t-shirt, feeling great and full of energy. The sun is shining, and life is good! Now write down your thoughts.

- See what's happening in your imagination.
- Be specific and vivid in your description.

This exercise will help you form your timeline and define your primary goal. As you're ready, try visualizing your life six months and one year from now.

Three months from now…

_____

_____

_____

Six months from now…

_____

_____

_____

One year from now…

_____

_____

_____

Once you have this vivid imagery in your head, you can increase your motivation by returning to it first thing in the morning, right before bed, and any time you're tempted by one of the Habits of Disease.

Keeping your focus on your primary choices will guide you through whatever life throws your way. We all have problems, but no matter how many we solve, there are always more to take their place. The point is, solving problems doesn't take you closer to your goal. That's why I spend most of my time focused on what I'm creating, whether it's a sailing trip with my family or simply getting to bed on time.

Let's go back to this exercise from lesson 3:

> Look down at the floor! (*your concepts*)
> Now look up at the ceiling! (*what you want*)
> Now, while looking up at the ceiling, can you see the floor?

Once you know where you are (your current reality), look up and stay focused on what you want to create (your primary choice, desire, or vision) rather than on the things you believe are wrong with you, your circumstances, your problems, and your self-limiting beliefs. When you put your time and effort into what you want, you'll experience a wonderful generative energy and start creating the life and health you desire. Now, I'm not saying you shouldn't address your problems, but give them just the energy they need and nothing more.

Let's say you have a burst water pipe. You turn off the water, clean the mess, and call the plumber. But instead of saying, "Well, my day is ruined now" and going for the potato chips, refocus on the choices that support your goals—one of which is a healthy weight. How about calling your husband, telling him there was a water line break and that the two of you are going out to dinner for a nice piece of fish and a salad!

The take-home message is it doesn't matter what you think you can or can't do or what's going on in your busy life. If you shift your focus to what's most important and put most of your energy to that end, you will make progress on the path to optimal health.

It's important to limit the effect that your concepts, beliefs, and problems have on your life, because these things can distract you from creating what you really want. Think of your concepts as a heavy stone you're holding onto while you tread water. You're exhausted, and soon you'll drown. But if you just let go of the rock (your concepts or self-limiting beliefs), you'll rise to the top and get what you want.

Giving recognition to a belief that's holding you back doesn't serve your ability to create what you want. By ceasing to give it energy, you'll begin to eliminate its influence

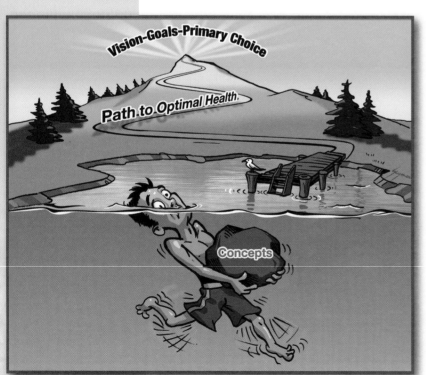

Vision-Goals-Primary Choice

Path to Optimal Health

Concepts

on your goal. Self-limiting beliefs simply don't have any place in the creative energy of structural tension. That's why we're going to practice shifting your focus to what's important and giving those things your undivided attention. Once you figure out what's most important to you, your primary and secondary choices will bring it into being. Let's see how this looks on our structural tension chart.

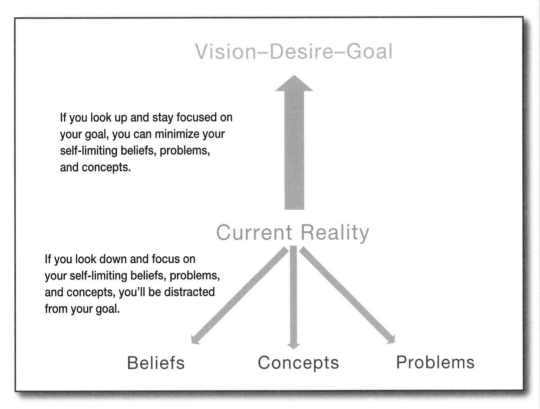

If you've made the choice of optimal health, your daily choices will reflect that and you won't be as inclined to give in to temptations that slow your progress. Now that you're on the path to health, what choices would you make?

MAKING CHOICES THAT LEAD YOU TO YOUR GOAL

CHOICE A	CHOICE B	YOUR CHOICE
Skip breakfast	Eat a healthy, low-calorie meal such as low-fat yogurt and strawberries with a cup of hot tea	_____ _____ _____ _____

Snack on a candy bar	Eat a piece of fruit or a protein bar	_____ _____
Sit around during lunch or your break	Walk around the building; climb a few flights of stairs; meditate; stretch; walk the dog	_____ _____ _____ _____
Save up calories for that big dinner	Eat every three hours; never skip a meal in order to eat more later	_____ _____ _____
Have a high-calorie, high-fat dessert	Have fruit, sorbet, coffee; have one bite and savor it	_____ _____
Go to happy hour	Run or go to the gym; play golf, tennis, or bike with friends	_____ _____
Choose fast food	Make your own meals or order salad with grilled chicken	_____ _____
Sit around being bored	Make a "to do" list and get your house, office, etc., in order	_____ _____ _____
Listen to negative self-talk	Read a positive book; review your goals	_____ _____
Stay up late watching TV and snacking	Go to bed early enough to get seven hours of sleep; tape your favorite late-night shows	_____ _____ _____ _____

Eat everything on your plate	Divide your plate into portions using the 1, 2, 3 rule from *Dr. A's Habits of Health*	_____
Drink soda or fruit drinks	Drink water (8–10 glasses daily)	_____
Eat 1–3 meals daily	Every three hours, eat a small low-glycemic, low-calorie, fuel-enhancing meal	_____
Shop when you're hungry, without a list	Shop after eating and stick to your list	_____
Drink alcohol	Have club soda with lime	_____
Reach for the snack cupboard	Sweep the front porch; take out two soup cans and use them for your weight-training exercises	_____
Try to get healthy alone	Ask a friend to join you; hire a health coach and trainer; join a gym	_____
Eat at a restaurant	Make your own healthy meals so you control how they're prepared	_____

I'll bet you're finding it much easier to make the right choices now that you're thinking in terms of goals rather than willpower! You're now equipped to learn the Habits of Health, and again I want to thank Robert Fritz for his mentorship, friendship, and contributions to the dynamics of creative process.

Section Two

The Habits of Reaching and Maintaining a Healthy Weight

LESSON 8 ▶ Reaching Your Healthy Weight

Take the first step on your path by learning how to safely get rid of unhealthy fat

BEFORE YOU BEGIN
Read Chapters 6 and 7 in *Dr. A's Habits of Health*

GOALS
- Understand the two core principles of weight loss through energy management
- Make your environment weight-loss ready
- Discover the importance of a keeping a journal and planning your day
- Learn how to use the catalyst for weight loss
- Get a handle on cravings
- Find out how to accelerate weight loss
- Create a structural tension chart for reaching a healthy weight

CREATE A NEW ENERGY MANAGEMENT SYSTEM

To reach and maintain a healthy weight, you need to take control of your energy management system—that is, calories in and calories out. It's also critical to get your body out of fat-storage mode and into fat-burning mode by controlling your body's release of insulin.

Take another look at the chart of our typical eating pattern on page 61 of *Dr. A's Habits of Health*. Does this resemble the way you eat? When we eat meals that are high in fat, sugar, and simple carbohydrates, our blood sugar and insulin levels increase and facilitate the accumulation of excess fat. This lesson is designed to help you fire your current energy management system and enter your new leptogenic world through a comprehensive approach that puts you in charge.

MAKE YOUR ENVIRONMENT WEIGHT-LOSS READY

Let's start your journey by making your world a place that supports your new Habits of Health. This is critical to your success, so make sure you complete these checklists *before* you go on to the next activity.

Kitchen makeover

As you learned in *Dr. A's Habits of Health,* one of your first steps is to learn proper portion size. Here are some tips:

- Put away your large plates and bowls and replace them with nine-inch plates and cup-size bowls. Use only small forks and spoons.
- Use a food scale and measuring cups to regulate portion size.
- Place the proper amount of food onto your plate in the kitchen and then leave the kitchen and sit in the dining room. Don't place serving dishes on the table that may tempt you to take a second helping.
- Consider painting your kitchen blue and using blue plates and placements. The color blue is known to decrease appetite while yellow and red increase it.
- Keep the lights on. Studies show that we tend to eat less in bright light.

Kitchen checklist

✓ Food scale
✓ Measuring cups
✓ Small cups and bowls
✓ 7- to 9-inch dinner plates
✓ Teaspoons and salad forks
✓ Blue placemats and plates
✓ Bright lights

Refrigerator and cupboard makeover

Make it easy to avoid high-calorie, high-fat meals and snacks by getting rid of the following:

- Whole-fat dairy products (whole milk, cheese, yogurt, cottage cheese, butter, and mayonnaise)
- Processed deli meats
- Fattening salad dressings
- White bread, pasta, rice, and flour
- Fruit drinks
- Cookies, pastries, desserts

Be sure you don't use this exercise as a last chance to eat all the Oreo cookies left in the bag! Instead, give foods away to a neighbor or food bank. Remember, once you get to your healthy weight, you can have an occasional Oreo if you want it.

Refrigerator and cupboard checklist
Now restock your fridge and cupboards with these*:

✓ Fat-free or low-fat dairy products (skim milk, low-fat yogurt, low-fat cheeses)
✓ Lean proteins (skinless chicken, turkey breast, fish)
✓ Whole-grain bread and pasta, brown rice
✓ Beans
✓ Fresh fruits and vegetables
✓ Olive oil, vinegar, spray-type salad dressings
✓ Herbs and spices

If necessary, choose one cupboard for other family members to use for their foods that aren't on your list. Better yet, ask them to join you in putting an end to unhealthy eating habits!

Healthy snacks
Replace high-calorie foods like peanuts and chips with fresh green vegetables and fruits (if your eating plan permits fruit). Here are some great low-calorie snacks:

Asparagus (1/2 cup = 18 cal, 3 carbs)	Radishes (1 oz = 8 cal, 2 carbs)
Broccoli (1 cup = 44 cal, 8 carbs)	Spinach (1 cup = 6 cal, 1 carb)
Sugar-free Jello (1 snack cup = 10 cal, 0 carbs)	Bouillon (1 cup = 10 cal, 1 carb)
Cauliflower (2 oz = 12 cal, 2 carbs)	Cucumber (1 cup = 15 cal, 3 carbs)
Celery (1 stalk = 6 cal, 1 carb)	Lettuce (1 cup = 2 cal, 0 carbs)
Dill pickle (1 = 4 cal, 1 carb)	Spinach (1 cup = 6 cal, 1 carb)

And remember, before you grab something to eat, make sure you're actually hungry and not just thirsty. Around 30 percent of the time, thirst is disguised as hunger. Try drinking a big glass of water and waiting ten minutes. Then rate your hunger on a scale of 1 to 5. You may not need that snack after all!

Bedroom makeover
Studies show that sleep is key not just to our overall health, but to our ability to lose and maintain weight. That's why it's so important to get at least seven hours of sleep a night (eight for men). Design your bedroom for relaxation by using light, calming colors like peach, yellow, or lavender, and relaxing scents. Stay away from late-night TV and read a motivational book instead, or write out your affirmations in your journal. Get rid of clutter both in your bedroom and in your closets by taking all those clothes that are too big for you to a consignment shop— and never look back!

You'll find more tips on getting a good night's sleep in Chapter 17 of *Dr. A's Habits of Health* and lesson 13 of this guide.

---

* If you've chosen to use the medically formulated meal replacement (PCMR) program—which I think is a great choice—some of the foods listed here will be restricted just until you reach your healthy weight and enter the transition and maintenance phase. Instead, you'll be stocking up on foods that fit the "lean and green" profile that you learned about in *Dr. A's Habits of Health.*

Bedroom checklist

✓ Remove your TV and tape late-night shows instead.

✓ Decorate with light colors.

✓ Bring your journal to bed for your evening entry.

✓ Keep your bedroom neat.

✓ Use scented candles or potpourri.

✓ Play calming music.

✓ Keep motivational books on your nightstand.

✓ Get at least seven hours of sleep nightly (eight for men).

PREPARE YOUR JOURNAL

Keeping a daily journal is a great way to go from mindless to mindful as you move toward optimal health. Tracking your daily intake, thoughts, successes, and failures helps you learn what works and where you're struggling. Whether you choose a fancy journal, a simple spiral notebook, or a blog, make sure you can carry it with you and write in it daily.

Here's a great way to begin.

Page One: Place your "before" picture.

Page Two: Write down your goal and the secondary choices that support that goal. You can use the detailed description you created in the last lesson.

First Page of Each Week: Write down a goal for the week, such as "I will eat a small, low-fat meal every three hours" or "I will wear my pedometer and take 5,000 extra steps every day this week." Give yourself a reward for reaching your weekly goal, such a fitness magazine, a book, or running shoes.

Each Week: Enter the following into your journal:

The times you eat	Types of exercise you enjoy
The foods you eat	The amount of weight lost that week
How much water you drink	How you feel before and after you eat
Any learning experiences	Better choices for next time (if applicable)

PLAN YOUR DAY

Daily planning helps you control your choices. Each day, prepare a schedule that determines when, where, and what you'll eat. Have a back-up plan in place for those days that just don't go as planned. I always carry a meal replacement bar or some kind of healthy food with me just in case I can't stop what I'm doing when it's time for a fueling.

It's a good idea to write out your plan the night before. Here's an example.

YOUR PLANNED DAY	TIME	YOUR ACTUAL DAY	TIME
Get up	6:30 am	_____	_____
Breakfast (oatmeal)	7:00 am	_____	_____
Exercise	7:30–8:30 am	_____	_____
At work (bottled water)	9:00 am	_____	_____
Snack (shake)	10:00 am	_____	_____
Lunch (soup)	12:30 pm	_____	_____
Snack (bar)	3:30 pm	_____	_____
Dinner (Lean and Green™)	6:30 pm	_____	_____
Snack (pudding)	9:30 pm	_____	_____
Sleep	10:30 pm	_____	_____

THE CATALYST TO RAPID WEIGHT LOSS

In Chapter 7 of *Dr. A's Habits of Health,* you learned about medically formulated portion-controlled meal replacements (PCMRs)—a very safe and effective way to start you on your way to losing unhealthy pounds and move you toward optimal health.

Before you begin, be sure to you've read that chapter and completed all the lessons in this workbook so far. Even if you're not on the PCMR plan, you'll benefit greatly by reading this section.

Your first three days may be a little challenging as your body ramps up its use of fat as an energy source. You'll also find that the rhythm of your day will change as you begin to focus less on food and its preparation. But once your body kicks into a fat-burning state, you'll feel great, have lots of energy, and your appetite will be noticeably reduced.

As you learned in Chapter 7, you'll be having five meal replacements and one Lean and Green meal each day. Be sure to write your daily routine out for the first two weeks until you really learn your new schedule. Remember to start your day with a meal replacement within an hour of waking up.

YOUR DAILY SCHEDULE

	TIME	MEAL	THOUGHTS
1.			
2.			
3.			
4.			
5.			
6.			
7.			

Amount of water: _____

You'll notice that I added an extra entry for a snack if needed. If you feel especially hungry (which may happen during the first few days) and the "free" food snacks aren't enough, it's fine to have another shake or soup. You'll still kick into the fat-burning state within the third or fourth day, and it will help you stay focused on the program and out of the cupboards!

A REVIEW OF YOUR LEAN AND GREEN FROM *DR. A'S HABITS OF HEALTH*

LEAN CHOICES

LIST SOME GOOD SEAFOOD CHOICES. (HOH page 79)

_____

_____

_____

_____

_____

LIST SOME GOOD MEAT AND POULTRY CHOICES. (HOH page 80)

_____

_____

_____

_____

_____

LIST SOME GOOD MEATLESS OPTIONS. (HOH page 80)

_____

_____

_____

_____

_____

GREEN VEGETABLE AND SALAD CHOICES

LIST SOME LOW-CARBOHYDRATE CHOICES. (HOH page 82)

_____

_____

_____

_____

_____

LIST SOME MODERATE-CARBOHYDRATE CHOICES. (HOH page 82)

LIST SOME HIGH-CARBOHYDRATE CHOICES. (HOH page 82)

LIST SOME SNACKS YOU'LL KEEP AVAILABLE AT HOME OR WORK. (HOH page 83)

LIST SOME HEALTHY FATS. (HOH page 81)

_____
_____
_____
_____
_____

LIST THE FIVE CRUCIAL DIETARY HABITS THAT WILL HELP YOU LOSE WEIGHT QUICKLY AND SAFELY. (HOH page 84)

1. _____
2. _____
3. _____
4. _____
5. _____

Now review the checklist on page 84 of _Dr. A's Habits of Health_ to make sure you're optimizing your weight-loss success.

The Habit of Health you've learned in this section is to fuel your body every three hours that you're awake.

WHAT WILL THIS HABIT DO FOR YOU? (HOH page 63)

_____
_____
_____
_____
_____
_____
_____

BEAT CRAVINGS

While most people lose their craving for sugar and other carbohydrates while on the program, they can still occur. Because most food cravings last less than fifteen minutes, it's a good idea to make a list of chores that take about that long—maybe cleaning out the sock drawer or the cupboard under the sink, straightening a room or your office, sweeping the porch or garage, or washing some windows. When you feel a craving, grab a big glass of water and choose one of the projects on your list. You'll walk away with a feeling of accomplishment *and* the knowledge that you stuck to your program!

Choosing an activity over eating is especially helpful when you're dealing with a stressful day and looking for comfort food. Get away from the area that's causing the stress and take a walk, listen to music, or choose from your chore list. It may also help to ask yourself whether the action you're contemplating supports your primary choice to reach a healthy weight.

WHAT ARE SOME ACTIVITIES YOU CAN DO AROUND THE HOUSE OR OFFICE WHEN YOU FEEL STRESS OR A CRAVING?

1. _____
2. _____
3. _____
4. _____
5. _____
6. _____
7. _____
8. _____
9. _____
10. _____

ACCELERATE YOUR WEIGHT LOSS

Here are some tips to enhance your progress on the meal-replacement plan:

1. Eat your first meal replacement within an hour of waking up.
2. Don't overexercise. If you haven't been exercising, don't start now. Wait three weeks. Then you can begin to add activity to your schedule as you learn Habits of Motion that are sustainable over time. If you're already exercising, cut the amount of weight you use by half and don't do more than 20 minutes of exercise a day for the first three weeks. No huffing, puffing, or sweating! After three weeks, you can add more weights and exercise, but while you're on this low-calorie program, don't exceed 45 minutes of moderate activity.
3. Be sure to have all five meal replacements and your lean and green meal each day. Eat slowly and use a straw for liquids.
4. Drink plenty of water. Divide your weight by two to find out how many ounces you should drink daily. (For example, if you weigh 220 pounds, you should drink 110 ounces of water per day.) *How much water should* you *drink?* _____ (Remember, you can also use iced tea or Crystal Light to satisfy your daily amount.)
5. Measure your lean and green meal portions and stick to them.
6. Keep your daily carbohydrate level between 85 and 100 grams, though 85 is optimal. Your lean and green meal should contain about 10 carbohydrates.
7. Take advantage of all the support you can, whether through meetings, chat rooms (positive ones only!), support calls, or a personal coach.
8. Keep your journal every day.
9. Review your goal and secondary choices every day.
10. Have no more than two approved snacks per day, if needed.
11. Don't add extra carbohydrates such as bread, pasta, rice, or fruit.
12. Don't drink alcohol of any sort.

The chart on the next page is just like the one you used in the previous chapter when you learned how to create a structural tension chart. Now that you have a better idea how to reach a healthy weight, you can modify your goals, time, and other adjustments as needed. If you have a lot of weight to lose, you may need to adjust the timeline. As a rough guide, the average person loses 2–5 lbs per week for the first two weeks, and 1–2 lbs per week thereafter. So, for example, if you're a man and need to lose thirty pounds to reach your healthy weight, it should take you about 12–16 weeks. If nothing has changed for you, just fill this chart in with the information you used in the last lesson. You'll be filling in these charts to help you reach all of the Habits of Health to come.

YOUR STRUCTURAL TENSION CHART FOR REACHING
A HEALTHY WEIGHT AND WAIST SIZE

Healthy Weight

Weight:
BMI:
Waist Circumference:

Secondary Choices

Timeline

1. Eating every three hours

2. _____

3. _____

4. _____

5. _____

6. _____

7. _____

8. _____

9. _____

_____

_____

_____

_____

_____

_____

Current Reality

Weight:
BMI:
Waist Circumference:

LESSON 9 ▸ Eating for Weight Control

Master calorie control and develop the Habits of Energy Management

BEFORE YOU BEGIN
Read Chapters 8, 9, and 10 in *Dr. A's Habits of Health*

GOALS
- Understand the two core principles of weight loss through energy management
- Discover Dr. A's system of weight control
- Learn how to use the nine-inch plate, three-component system, and color-coded shopping system
- Determine how your daily schedule will look as you reach your ideal weight
- Create a structural tension chart for reaching a healthy weight

---

IN THE LAST LESSON, YOU LEARNED THE TWO KEY COMPONENTS OF ENERGY MANAGEMENT AND WEIGHT LOSS:

1. _____

2. _____

These two principles—controlling your calorie intake and eating foods that don't turn on your insulin pump—are the secrets to a long-term eating strategy that will keep you thriving throughout your longer, healthier life.

In addition, the following three simple tools will help you create portion-controlled, low-glycemic, lower-calorie fuelings for every meal—whether you're eating at a restaurant, on the run, or at home.

1. **The nine-inch plate system** creates instant portion control.
2. **The three-component system** helps you master correct servings of meat, starches, and vegetables by using familiar visuals for sizing—a deck of cards, a tennis ball, and a small paperback book.
3. **The color charts** provide an easy system to use when you're shopping for food. Stay in the green and stay lean!

THE NINE-INCH PLATE AND THREE-COMPONENT SYSTEMS

Learn this system and you'll soon be able to control your portion size whether you're at home or out.

LIST THE THREE VITAL MACRONUTRIENTS. (HOH page 152)

1. _____

2. _____

3. _____

LIST THE THREE MAJOR FOOD GROUPS. (HOH page 89)

1. _____

2. _____

3. _____

Which food group should make up half your plate? (HOH page 89)

_____

Which two food groups should make up the other half? (HOH page 89)

_____

How many calories should you eat per day while you work on those last few pounds? (HOH page 90) _____

FILL IN THE NINE-INCH PLATE
WITH THE PROPER FOOD GROUPS.

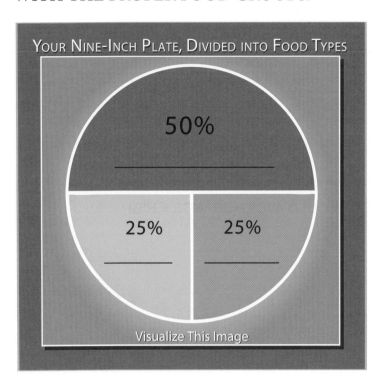

YOUR NINE-INCH PLATE, DIVIDED INTO FOOD TYPES

50%

_____

25%

_____

25%

_____

Visualize This Image

THE COLOR-CODED SHOPPING SYSTEM

To answer the following questions, refer to the color-coded charts in Chapter 9 of *Dr. A's Habits of Health*.

1. Starches
Starches are a wonderful slow-burning fuel, rich in fiber and vitamin B, calcium, potassium, and phosphorus. In their natural form, they're also low glycemic.

Look for starches with a glycemic index of less than _____. (HOH page 107)

The portion of starch on your plate should be about the size of _____. (HOH page 107)

LIST SOME HEALTHY STARCHES (GREEN = LOW GLYCEMIC). (HOH page 107)

1. _____
2. _____
3. _____
4. _____

LIST SOME HIGH-GLYCEMIC STARCHES YOU SHOULD AVOID (ORANGE = HIGH GLYCEMIC). (HOH page 107)

1. _____
2. _____
3. _____
4. _____
5. _____

2. Protein

Protein is a basic building block for all your vital organs and tissue. It's critical during weight loss to protect your muscle and provide new building material for your continuous renewal process. Protein also helps to suppress hunger.

The portion of protein on your plate should be about the size of _____. (HOH page 109)

LIST SOME HEALTHY PROTEIN CHOICES. (HOH page 100–102)

1. _____
2. _____
3. _____
4. _____
5. _____

LIST SOME HIGH-FAT MEATS YOU SHOULD AVOID. (HOH page 102)

1. _____
2. _____
3. _____

3. Fruits and Vegetables

Fruits and vegetables are an excellent source of vitamins, minerals, and phytonutrients. They're also full of fiber, which provides bulk and fills you up.

The portion of fruits and vegetables on your plate should be about the size of _____

_____. (HOH page 98)

LIST SOME HEALTHY FRUITS (DARK GREEN = VERY LOW GLYCEMIC). (HOH page 100)

1. _____
2. _____
3. _____
4. _____
5. _____

LIST SOME POOR FRUIT CHOICES (RED = HIGH GLYCEMIC). (HOH page 100)

1. _____
2. _____
3. _____
4. _____
5. _____

LIST SOME HEALTHY VEGETABLES (DARK GREEN = VERY LOW GLYCEMIC). (HOH page 99)

1. _____
2. _____
3. _____
4. _____
5. _____

LIST SOME POOR VEGETABLE CHOICES (ORANGE = HIGH GLYCEMIC). (HOH page 99)

1. _____
2. _____
3. _____
4. _____
5. _____

4. Fats

The majority of fat in our Western diet is extremely unhealthy. It comes from_____ and is mostly _____ fat. (HOH page 109)

Saturated fat derives from animals and is found in high levels in hot dogs, hamburgers, bacon, and fatty meats.

Hydrogenated fats are used to extend the shelf life of many foods and are known as _____ _____. (HOH page 110) Their ingestions is directly linked to vessel plaque formation, heart attacks, and strokes.

I recommend you limit fat to 20–25 percent of your daily caloric intake, with no more than 5 percent from saturated fat. As a Habit of Health, you should have no more than _____ grams of saturated fat per day. (HOH page 111)

Butter is full of saturated fat, and margarine is full of trans-fat. Name a form of margarine that is free of trans-fats: _____ (HOH page 111, sidebar)

Healthy fats help turn off insulin, help unload triglycerides from fat cells, increase your metabolism, and protect your muscle membranes. These healthy fats, known as essential fatty acids or omega fats, represent a Habit of Health and should be part of your daily diet.

LIST SOME SOURCES OF HEALTHY FATS. (HOH page 112, sidebar)

1. _____

2. _____

3. _____

4. _____

5. Legumes

Legumes include a wide variety of beans, peas, and lentils. They're inexpensive, packed with nutrients, and contain lots of fiber, which makes them a natural cholesterol-lowering food. They're also low glycemic, which helps turn off your insulin pump.

LIST SOME HEALTHY LEGUMES. (HOH page 104)

1. _____

2. _____

3. _____

4. _____

5. _____

6. Water

Water is a critical component of your body, making up between 55 and 60 percent of your weight. Optimum hydration is essential to the proper functioning of your organs and systems. It's the solvent that moves nutrients, hormones, antibodies, and oxygen through your bloodstream and lymphatic system. It also helps remove waste and toxins from your body.

Adults lose nearly _____ 8-ounce cups of water daily. (HOH page 114) That's 96 ounces of loss per day!

To find out how many ounces of water you should have daily, divide your weight by two:

Your weight _____ divided by 2 = _____ ounces of water per day

To review more reasons to drink water, see page 114 of *Dr. A's Habits of Health,* and remember this Habit of Health:

Drink a glass of water on rising and before each meal.

YOUR HEALTHY EATING SCHEDULE

While you're reaching your healthy weight, an average day's fueling should like this (fill in the time of day):

TIME	MEAL	CALORIES
_____	Breakfast	300–400
_____	Mid-morning	100
_____	Lunch	100–200
_____	Mid-afternoon	100
_____	Dinner	400
_____	Evening	100

LIST SOME OF YOUR 100–CALORIE FUELING CHOICES. (HOH pages 120–121)

1. _____
2. _____
3. _____
4. _____
5. _____

LIST SOME OF YOUR 300–400 CALORIE BREAKFAST CHOICES. (HOH pages 122–128)

1. _____
2. _____
3. _____
4. _____
5. _____

LIST SOME OF YOUR 100–200 CALORIE LUNCH CHOICES. (HOH pages 122–128)

1. _____
2. _____
3. _____
4. _____
5. _____

LIST SOME OF YOUR 400-CALORIE DINNER CHOICES. (HOH pages 122–128)

1. _____
2. _____
3. _____
4. _____
5. _____

YOUR STRUCTURAL TENSION CHART FOR REACHING A HEALTHY WEIGHT AND WAIST SIZE USING DR. A'S HEALTHY EATING SYSTEM

Healthy Weight

Weight:
BMI:
Waist Circumference:

Secondary Choices

Timeline

1. Eating every three hours

2. _____ _____

3. _____ _____

4. _____

5. _____ _____

6. _____ _____

7. _____

8. _____ _____

9. _____ _____

Current Reality

Weight:
BMI:
Waist Circumference:

LESSON 10 ▸ Eating Healthy for Life

Discover foods and eating habits that will optimize your health for life

BEFORE YOU BEGIN
Read Chapters 11 and 12 in *Dr. A's Habits of Health*

GOALS
- Understand the core habits of weight control
- Find out why reaching your healthy weight is just the beginning
- Calculate your set point for adding calories
- Discover healthy vs. unhealthy food choices
- Learn how to manage your hunger
- Transition to healthy eating for life
- Create a structural tension chart for mastering the BeSlim™ lifestyle

Now that you're on your way to reaching your optimal weight and learning the Habits of Health that will sustain you for life, let's review the core habits for maintaining a healthy weight from Chapters 11 and 12 of *Dr. A's Habits of Health*.

THE BESLIM LIFESTYLE

You've now learned the six beginning habits for maintaining a healthy weight. I've created an acronym to help you remember them: BeSlim.

WHAT DOES BESLIM STAND FOR? (HOH page 149)

B _____

E _____

S _____

L _____

I _____

M _____

Make sure you understand these key habits thoroughly by reviewing pages 149–151 in *Dr. A's Habits of Health*. You should also be applying them to your structural tension chart. Fully embracing these core habits is critical to maintaining a healthy weight.

There are two main reasons that diets fail: first, a lack of understanding of energy balance, and second, a lack of proper motivation, which you learned about in lessons 5 and 6.

EXPLAIN WHAT A CLASSIC YO-YO DIET PATTERN IS AND HOW IT OCCURS.
(HOH page 151)

_____

_____

_____

_____

_____

Remember, reaching your healthy weight is only the first step in attaining optimal health and a longer life. To transition from weight loss to a lifetime strategy of eating healthy for life you need to focus on two key areas (HOH page 153):

1. Adding calories until_____

2. Introducing a full range of_____

As you'll recall from Chapter 12 of *Dr. A's Habits of Health*, your *set point* is the point at which the number of calories you take in is equal to the number of calories you use, and it's the key to maintaining your weight. Take care not to overshoot this number, or you'll regain weight as you add more food groups and increase your intake.

Let's start figuring out your set point by calculating your Total Energy Expenditure (TEE).

TOTAL ENERGY EXPENDITURE (ENERGY OUT)

WHAT THREE FACTORS ADDED TOGETHER DETERMINE YOUR TEE? (HOH page 154)

1. _____

2. _____

3. _____

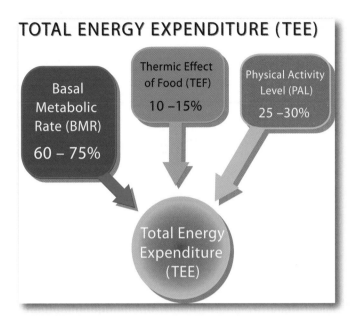

TOTAL ENERGY EXPENDITURE (TEE)

In *Dr. A's Habits of Health,* we present two different ways to calculate your TEE and determine a starting point for figuring out how many calories you're currently burning. Let's review the simpler method here.

Your current weight (in pounds) x 11 calories = your TEE (daily caloric need)

Your TEE: _____

Now, adjust your TEE to take into account your current activity level. To do so, multiply your TEE by:

　　　1.2 for light exercise
　　　1.5 for moderate exercise
　　　1.7 for heavy exercise

For example: 162 lbs x 11 kcal/lb = 1,782 kcal x 1.2 = 2,138 kcal/day

Your TEE = _____ lbs x 11 kcal/lb = _____kcal x _____ = _____kcal/day

Remember to adjust your TEE as your weight and activity level change.

Transitioning to your permanent eating plan can be as easy as adding about 100 calories to your daily intake each week until you reach your TEE.

How many weeks will it take to reach your set point (TEE)? _____ (HOH page 161)

Use the following structural tension chart to help you transition to your healthy set point. (You may need to use fewer or more weeks than are on the chart.)

YOUR STRUCTURAL TENSION CHART FOR REACHING YOUR TEE

Your Calculated TEE (kcal)

_____

Timeline (weeks)

_____ kcal
_____ kcal
_____ kcal
_____ kcal
_____ kcal
_____ kcal
_____ kcal
_____ kcal
_____ kcal
_____ kcal

Current Calorie Intake _____

Current Reality

FOOD CHOICES FOR WEIGHT MAINTENANCE

LIST THE THREE CORE PRINCIPLES FOR REACHING AND MAINTAINING A HEALTHY WEIGHT. (HOH page 131)

1. _____

2. _____

3. _____

Now let's take each of these core principles and relate them to real life.

LIST SOME METHODS FOR MASTERING CALORIES IN. (HOH page 131–132)

1. _____

2. _____

3. _____

LIST THE THREE MAJOR MACRONUTRIENTS USED FOR FUEL. (HOH page 132)

1. _____
2. _____
3. _____

WHY IS IT BETTER TO EAT LOW-GLYCEMIC FOODS? (HOH page 134)

_____
_____
_____
_____
_____

WHAT CORE PRINCIPLES SHOULD YOU USE TO CONTROL YOUR HUNGER?
(HOH page 138)

1. _____
2. _____
3. _____
4. _____
5. _____

LIST SOME LOW-DENSITY FOODS THAT YOU CAN ENJOY. (HOH page 139)

1. _____
2. _____
3. _____
4. _____

LIST SOME HIGH-DENSITY FOODS THAT YOU SHOULD AVOID. (HOH page 139)

1. _____

2. _____

3. _____

4. _____

The best and most efficient way to remove excess visceral adiposity (fat) is through: (HOH page 142)

_____Exercise

_____Producing a fat-burning state

As you transition to your lifelong eating plan, review pages 158–166 in *Dr. A's Habits of Health* to help you choose your foods wisely.

YOUR STRUCTURAL TENSION CHART TO GUIDE YOUR TRANSITION

Your Calculated TEE (kcal)

_____

Adding food groups (if using PCMR)	Timeline (weeks)

Week 4 _____

Week 3 _____

Week 2 _____

Week 1 _____

_____ kcal
_____ kcal
_____ kcal
_____ kcal
_____ kcal
_____ kcal
_____ kcal
_____ kcal
_____ kcal
_____ kcal

Current Calorie Intake _____

Current Reality

PREPARING FOR TRANSITION: ARE YOU READY?

1. Once you've reached your healthy weight, you can…
   a. Eat whatever you like
   b. Eat only fruits and vegetables
   c. Gradually add calories from all the food groups
   d. Stop exercising. You've made it!

2. Transition is a great time to add high-quality proteins, nutrient-dense starches, and a variety of low-glycemic fruits and vegetables to your diet.

LIST SOME HEALTHY EATING STRATEGIES THAT WILL HELP YOU ALONG THE WAY.
(HOH page 162)

a. _____

b. _____

c. _____

d. _____

e. _____

f. _____

---

3. Berries are very low glycemic and a good choice. T / F

4. Corn and peas are examples of low-glycemic vegetables. T / F

5. Which potato is the best choice?
   a. white
   b. sweet
   c. yams

5. Which of these types of bread is a healthy choice?
   a. pumpernickel
   b. white wheat
   c. sourdough
   d. whole wheat
   e. all of the above except b

6. Commercial breakfast cereals are a wise choice. T / F

7. Rice is very high glycemic and should only be eaten occasionally and in small amounts. T /F

8. You should eat red meat at least three times a week. T/ F

9. Your permanent eating strategies should include meals that have five qualities:

LIST THE FIVE QUALITIES YOUR MEALS SHOULD HAVE. (HOH page 150)

a. _____

b. _____

c. _____

d. _____

e. _____

EATING HEALTHY WHEN DINING OUT

Become a master at eating out by learning what's healthy and what isn't. Here's a brief review of the recommendations on pages 166–169 of *Dr. A's Habits of Health.*

- Avoid fast food restaurants and all-you-can-eat buffets.
- Avoid alcohol, which is full of empty calories.
- If you want a cocktail, make it a small glass (5 oz) of red wine.
- Order your meal before you order a cocktail.
- Ask for the bread and/or chips to be removed from the table.
- Bring your own low-calorie dressing or ask for vinegar and oil to make your own.
- Stay away from scampi-style and au gratin dishes and from grilled or blackened meats. These are usually high in fat and dripping in butter.
- Choose dishes that are baked, grilled, poached, or steamed (or broiled if it's listed as a "light" dish).
- Choose lean cuts of meats and remove the skin from chicken before eating.
- Have the chef trim excess fat off your meat before cooking.
- Ask for vegetables to be steamed with no added butter or sugar.
- Visualize the nine-inch plate.
- Order two appetizers instead of an entrée.
- Split a meal with your companion.
- Ask for a leftover container at the beginning of the meal. Keep a proper portion on your plate and put the rest in the container for another time.

You now have the experience and knowledge to make a difference in your health and your life. Soon people will notice your new body, your increased energy, and your love of life—and you'll be a great inspiration to so many others who need to know what you know!

YOUR STRUCTURAL TENSION CHART
FOR MASTERING THE BESLIM LIFESTYLE

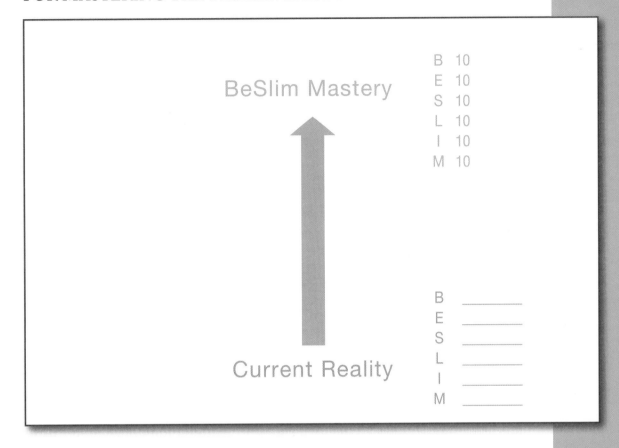

LESSON 11 ▸ Habits of Active Living

Burn calories for long-term weight control without taking time from your busy schedule through this easy, progressive plan

BEFORE YOU BEGIN
Read Chapters 13 to 15 in *Dr. A's Habits of Health*

GOALS
- Understand how energy-saving devices are robbing you of your health
- Discover the importance of increasing your energy expenditure
- Learn the NEAT System
- Prepare for the program by seeing your primary care physician
- Obtain tools for success
- Find your current level of NEAT
- Start your NEAT program
- Create a structural tension chart for burning calories through NEAT

In today's world, we're all so busy that any electronic device, machine, or shortcut that makes our daily tasks less effortful becomes ever more desirable. But while these tools do provide comfort and ease to our lifestyles, they're also robbing us of our health. Who would have thought that a remote control or automatic dishwasher had such power?

We humans are no longer active enough to support a healthy level of energy expenditure and keep our cardiovascular and musculoskeletal systems healthy. And yet, trying to use exercise as a substitute for an active lifestyle fails for most of us—first, because there are so many barriers to exercise (see page 178 in *Dr. A's Habits of Health*), and second, because for those of us who are overweight or obese, exercise may be too challenging and may even put us at risk (see page 170 in *Dr. A's Habits of Health*).

The good news is that you are now at an important crossroads that offers you the perfect opportunity to learn a simple, sustainable movement plan.

BEFORE YOU BEGIN

Consult your doctor before starting the Habits of Motion program. This is particularly important if you've lost a lot of weight and have been previously inactive. I recommend a complete physical that takes into account any pre-existing health conditions such as knee or joint problems, arthritis, or high blood pressure. Be sure to discuss with your doctor how these conditions may be affected by an increase in movement.

DR. A'S HABITS OF MOTION PART 1: THE NEAT SYSTEM

Do you use a remote control, make meals with electric devices instead of manual ones, slouch in that comfy desk chair at work, or use the restroom nearest to your office?

Of course you do!

Many of use have unintentionally become slaves to luxury—and who can blame us? Luxury, at first glance, seems desirable. But in reality, feeding our biological programming and conserving energy at a time when we can ill afford to do so has led us to fatigue, obesity, and illness. We need activity to maintain our musculoskeletal and cardiovascular systems, and to sustain the energy balance that prevents weight gain. The scientific term for this is *activity thermogenesis,* and every movement counts—even standing up and walking to the TV to change the channel instead of using the remote!

But together, we're going to morph your regular daily activities into an efficient system that will help you expend more energy and enjoy lasting health.

My NEAT System provides a simple and painless way to burn calories without disrupting your daily schedule or requiring vigorous effort. Here's how:

1. It provides an easy-to-do movement plan that's safe and effective for anyone, even if you've been overweight or inactive.
2. It will help you expend an additional 100–200 calories to offset the decrease in TEE you're experiencing as you lose body mass through weight loss.
3. It enables you to tap into all 168 hours in the week in ways that are sustainable for a lifetime of health.

YOUR NEAT SYSTEM GOALS

To set your NEAT System goals, you first need to establish your baseline of activity by doing the following:

- Read "Before You Begin" on page 193 of *Dr. A's Habits of Health.*
- Make copies of the Daily NEAT Activity Log, Weekly NEAT Activity Log, and NEAT Scoring Sheet available in Appendix A or at www.habitsofhealth.net.
- For seven days, use the logs to track your NEAT activities from the time you get up until

you hit the pillow at night. This will give you a valuable baseline—and support your primary choice to maintain a healthy weight!

Once you've monitored and recorded your first seven days, it's time to set some goals. You want to work toward 120 NEAT points per day for the next thirty days. Let's see how you're going to get there.

THE SIX S'S OF SUCCESS

Remember these activities from Chapter 15 of *Dr. A's Habits of Health*?

Stance

Standing

Strolling

Stairs

Samba

Switch

Which one appeals to you most? _____

HOW CAN I REALISTICALLY INCORPORATE THIS ACTIVITY INTO MY DAILY LIFE?
(HOH pages 188–193)

1. _____
2. _____
3. _____
4. _____
5. _____

WHAT BARRIERS MAY HINDER ME? (HOH pages 188–193)

1. _____
2. _____
3. _____
4. _____
5. _____

HOW WILL I OVERCOME THESE BARRIERS? (HOH pages 188–193)

1. _____
2. _____
3. _____
4. _____
5. _____

PUTTING YOUR PLAN IN MOTION

Before you begin, make sure you have the following tools at hand:

1. Heart-rate monitor
2. Stopwatch
3. Pedometer
4. NEAT Goal Setter (available in Appendix B or at www.habitsofhealth.net).

Complete the previous written exercises for each of the Six S's of Success—then put your plan into action today! Be sure to use your Daily NEAT Activity Log to document each time you improve your Stance, Standing, Strolling, Stairs, Samba, and Switch. After thirty days, review your NEAT Activity Log.

I think you'll find that not only is this system easy to do, it's actually a lot of fun! And best of all, making these secondary choices to incorporate the Six S's of Success into your day will support your healthy weight and a lifetime of health.

YOUR STRUCTURAL TENSION CHART FOR BURNING CALORIES THROUGH NEAT

NEAT Additional Calorie Expenditure

Secondary Choices   **Timeline**

Stance   _____

Standing   _____

Strolling   _____

Stairs   _____

Samba   _____

Switch   _____

Baseline _____

Current Reality

Your Goal:
- 120 NEAT Points (calories) per day for the first 30 days
- 200 NEAT Points (calories) per day for the second 30 days

LESSON 12 ▸ Muscles in Motion

Support and maintain healthy muscles in just thirty minutes a day

BEFORE YOU BEGIN
Read Chapter 16 in *Dr. A's Habits of Health*

GOALS
- Learn the three key goals of the Habits of Motion
- Start and progress through the EAT Walking Program
- Start the EAT Resistance Program
- Create a structural tension chart for the EAT programs

NEAT's pretty neat, isn't it? As you've now discovered, every movement makes a difference, and you've seen firsthand how enhancing your normal, everyday activities cranks up your thermogeneis.

Let's keep that momentum going through the EAT Walking Program, which will help you achieve the three core goals of the Habits of Motion by:

- Increasing your energy expenditure
- Optimizing your cardiovascular health
- Building a strong, healthy support system of bones and muscles

NOTE: Before you begin the EAT programs, be sure that you're comfortable with NEAT, have lost weight, have consulted with your doctor, and understand how to stay safe (see pages 198–199 in *Dr. A's Habits of Health*).

Now, as you continue to maintain and gradually increase your NEAT, you're going to begin to incorporate the EAT Walking Program into your daily activities to produce fitness. But please take your time! Slow and steady progress will help you learn more about your body and maximize your results.

THE EAT WALKING PROGRAM

Day One: Where Are You Today?

First, let's get a better picture of your current state of health and create an action plan to move you toward an increased level of fitness.

Step One

Do you have the following readily available?

- ❑ Comfortable, breathable workout clothes
- ❑ Comfortable, supportive walking shoes
- ❑ A pedometer
- ❑ A safe route to walk
- ❑ Time available in your day to walk for 20–30 minutes, five days a week

If not, your first assignment is to make sure you do before you move on to step two.

Step Two

What's your target heart rate? (See page 184 in *Dr. A's Habits of Health.*)

1. 220 – your age = _____ or your maximum heart rate.
2. Take your answer to question one and multiply it by 0.5. This will give you the minimum desirable beats per minute (BPM) as we start your conditioning.
3. Now take your answer to question one and multiply it by 0.65. This is the maximum beats per minute (BPM) as we start your conditioning.

Ideally, you should stay between these numbers until you feel comfortable with more intense exercise.

Your target heart rate is between _____ BPM and _____BPM.

Step Three

LIST ANY PROBLEM AREAS THAT REQUIRE STRETCHING PRIOR TO EXERCISE.

_____

_____

_____

_____

_____

Be sure to properly stretch each area once you've warmed up. (See page 201 in *Dr. A's Habits of Health.*)

> ### *Important Rules for Stretching*
>
> - The best time to stretch is directly after your walk.
> - Never stretch cold muscles.
> - Problem areas may be stretched prior to your walk, but only after you've warmed up.
> - Don't bounce when you stretch.
> - Ease into a stretch slowly and hold gently. Stretch to the point where you feel a gentle pull, but never to the point of pain.
> - Hold each stretch for 30 to 40 seconds. If you have problems with a particular area, stretch that area twice. (Hold for 30 to 40 seconds, release, then stretch again.)

Step Four

Ready, set, walk! Now that you have your gear, have identified your target BPM, and know what areas need special attention when stretching, you're ready to walk. Here's a goal to set for your initial walking sessions. You can use either the amount of time or the number of steps to keep track.

Warm up	5 minutes at 1 mph (about 160 steps)
Stretch problem areas	
Moderate pace	10 minutes at 2 mph (about 665 steps)
Cool down	5 minutes at 1 mph (about 160 steps)
Stretch	

Step Five

Enter the day's information on the EAT Walking Program Daily Tracking Sheet (available in Appendix B or at www.habitsofhealth.net).

Step Six

Next to day one on you EAT Walking Program Daily Tracking Sheet, note your rate of perceived exertion (RPE) and your BPM.

If you find that your RPE is higher than 5 or your BPM is above your target heart rate, adjust as needed for tomorrow by walking slower or reducing the duration of your session. Remember, slow and steady wins the race!

If, on the other hand, you find that your RPE is lower than 3 or your BPM is below your target heart rate, you may want to pick up the pace a bit—while still taking care to avoid overexertion.

Step Seven

Continue steps four to six for the remainder of the week. At the end of the week, log your progress on the EAT Walking Program Weekly Tracking Sheet (available in Appendix B or at www.habitsofhealth.net).

RATE OF PERCEIVED EXERTION	
Borg Scale	RPE
0	nothing at all
0.5	very, very light
1	very light
2	light
3	moderate
4	somewhat hard
5 – 6	hard
7 – 8	very hard
9	very, very hard
10	maximum exertion

Week Two: Pick Up the Pace

On day one of week two, try to increase the intensity of your workout by adding five minutes to your moderate pace. Your workout this week will look like this:

Warm up	5 minutes at 1 mph (about 160 steps)
Stretch problem areas	
Moderate pace	15 minutes at 2 mph (about 665 steps)
Cool down	5 minutes at 1 mph (about 160 steps)
Stretch	

Now repeat steps five to seven from week one.

Week Three: From 5,000 to 20,000 Steps

Your goal each week is to add five minutes of moderate walking (3 to 4 miles per hour), until you're walking five days a week for thirty minutes each day. That's around 20,000 steps, or ten miles a week.

When you add the 200 calories you're burning through NEAT each day to your Energetic Step Value from the chart below, you'll find that you're using quite a number of calories. Exciting, isn't it?

ENERGETIC STEP VALUE (ESV)		
		(steps required to burn 1 kcal)
Body Mass Index BMI	ESV (Female)	ESV (Male)
18 – 24.9 Healthy	36 steps per kcal	28 steps per kcal
25 – 29.9 Overweight	30 steps per kcal	24 steps per kcal
30 – 34.9 Class I Obesity	24 steps per kcal	20 steps per kcal
35 – 39.9 Class II Obesity	18 steps per kcal	16 steps per kcal
Over 40 Class III Obesity	12 steps per kcal	11 steps per kcal

If you want to add intensity to your workout, review the tips on page 203 of *Dr. A's Habits of Health*. Now, keep up the great work, and when you've reached 20,000 steps a week and are ready, you can move on to the EAT Resistance Program.

YOUR STRUCTURAL TENSION CHART
FOR THE EAT WALKING PROGRAM

EAT Walking Program:
_____
_____

Secondary Choices

Timeline

1. Proper walking shoes

2. Pedometer

3. Stretching

4. _____

5. _____

6. _____

7. _____

8. _____

9. _____

Current Steps _____

Current Reality

Your goal each week is to add five minutes of moderate walking (3 to 4 miles per hour), until you're walking five days a week for thirty minutes each day. That's around 20,000 steps, or ten miles a week.

THE EAT RESISTANCE PROGRAM

Congratulations! You've incorporated the Six S's of Success through NEAT and have reached your goal of 20,000 steps a week through the EAT Walking Program. You're well on your way to optimal health. Your cardiovascular health is increasing, and your energy expenditure is amplified. Now, lets turn to your muscles and bones.

Sarcopenia—*a degeneration of muscle mass and strength, sometimes referred to as osteoporosis of the muscles—is a serious condition that affects people who don't use their muscles regularly for lifting and moving (see page 197 in* Dr. A's Habits of Health).

Adding the EAT Resistance Program to your weekly routine enables you to combat sarcopenic muscles. Now don't get me wrong, you won't look like a body builder through this program. But you will recondition and increase your muscles in both size and number.

Now, on the two days each week that you're not walking through the EAT Walking Program, you'll do thirty minutes of resistance exercise. Make sure those aren't two consecutive days. It's important to let your body recover for two days between workouts.

In Chapter 16 of *Dr. A's Habits of Health*, you learned the core principles of the EAT Resistance Program:

- Muscle groups are moved slowly through the full range of motion in order to eliminate gravity and momentum and work muscles more completely. *Improves strength, bone density and overall function.*
- Movements are held at the point of maximum contraction just before lock-out to enable the muscles to grow fatigued and encourage them to recruit more muscle fibers. *Builds muscle.*
- Focus is on the core muscles. *Improves overall stance and posture and maximizes energy expenditure.*
- Movement is continuous. *Boosts cardiovascular health.*
- Muscles are stretched to the full range of motion after each muscle-group movement. *Promotes long-term flexibility.*

Day One: Plan Your Program
Step One
Do you have the following readily available?
- ❑ Comfortable, breathable workout clothes
- ❑ Comfortable, supportive walking shoes
- ❑ A mat and stability ball
- ❑ A safe and spacious workout area
- ❑ Time available in your day to exercise for 20–30 minutes, two days a week

If not, your first assignment is to make sure you do before you move on to step two.

Step Two

LIST SOME WARM-UPS THAT INTEREST YOU. (See page 207 of *Dr. A's Habits of Health* for some examples.)

_____

_____

_____

_____

Step Three
Identify which area you'd like to work on first.

Upper body	Lower body
Core (upper)	Core (lower)
Chest	Thighs
Latissimus dorsi (back)	Gluteals
Shoulders	Hamstrings
Arms	Calves

Step Four

LIST FIVE EXERCISES YOU'D LIKE TO TRY that concentrate on the area of the body you've chosen to work on first. You'll find examples in Appendix E of *Dr. A's Habits of Health.* (Note: You don't have to use dumbbells in the beginning, but over time you may choose to enhance your workout with them, as well as with other tools such as medicine balls, a vest weight, and ankle weights.)

Step Five
- Begin each exercise with a slow, consistent contraction (eight seconds), hold in place just before lock-out (four seconds), then relax the muscle as you slowly return to your starting position (eight seconds)—for a total of twenty seconds per exercise.
- Immediately begin another repetition, for a total of five per exercise.
- Rest for twenty seconds after your five repetitions.

Step Six
Repeat step five for the remaining four exercises.

Step Seven
Once you've completed your five exercises, take five minutes to stretch the muscles groups you've just worked.

Step Eight

Log your workout on the corresponding Eat Resistance Program Training Log (available in Appendix B or at www.habitsofhealth.net).

Day Two: The Second Area

On your second day of the EAT Resistance Program, you'll work the other area of your body. Be sure it's been two days since your last EAT Resistance Program workout.

Repeat steps two through eight.

Week Two: Add Rotations

Add one extra rotation to your program. Adding rotations gradually in this way helps ensure that you understand and are benefiting from each exercise fully.

You've now increased your energy expenditure, activity thermogenesis, physical activity level, and basal metabolic rate—all in thirty minutes a day! Over time, you'll continue to reap the benefits of these newfound habits of motion.

YOUR STRUCTURAL TENSION CHART FOR THE EAT RESISTANCE PROGRAM

EAT Resistance Program:
_____
_____

Secondary Choices

1. _____
2. _____
3. _____
4. _____
5. _____
6. _____
7. _____
8. _____
9. _____

Timeline

_____
_____
_____
_____
_____
_____
_____
_____

Current Steps _____

Current Reality

LESSON 13 ▸ The Discipline of Healthy Sleep

Rejuvenate and reward your body with these secrets for restful sleep

BEFORE YOU BEGIN
Read Chapter 17 in *Dr. A's Habits of Health*

GOALS
- Understand the importance of sleep
- Track the quantity and quality of your sleep
- Evaluate and optimize the hours you sleep
- Evaluate and optimize the quality of your sleep
- Optimize your sleep environment and routine
- Create a structural tension chart for healthy sleep

Learning good sleep habits is just as important as learning habits of healthy eating and motion. And just like those other habits, improving your sleep requires your active participation and commitment.

Sleep helps restore organ function, stabilizes chemical imbalance, refreshes areas of the brain that control mood and behavior, replenishes nutrients, and repairs brain circuitry. And those are just some of the benefits. So you can see that the saying "You can sleep when you're dead" is dead wrong!

Sleep is essential in helping our bodies bounce back from the stress and pollutants of daily life. It even assists with healthy weight management.

Are you getting enough good-quality sleep? If not, here's a step-by-step process that will help.

PART ONE: HOW MUCH SLEEP DO YOU GET?

If you haven't yet done so, complete the Sleep Assessment on page 216 of *Dr. A's Habits of Health.* As you'll recall, women should get between six and seven hours of sleep each night, and men should get between seven and eight hours.

Are you clocking in enough hours of sleep? _____

If you're not, continue with part one. If you're already getting enough hours, skip to part two.

You may tend to go to bed earlier or wake up later in order to get the sleep you need. This determines your chronotype.

What is your chronotype? _____ (HOH page 217)

Remember, sleep is not a luxury!

HOW CAN YOU MODIFY YOUR SCHEDULE TO ENSURE THAT YOU GET ENOUGH SLEEP?

_____

_____

_____

_____

_____

_____

PART TWO: TRACK YOUR SLEEP QUALITY

You now know how much sleep you need and have modified your schedule to make sure you get in enough hours. But how do you know that the sleep you're getting is really giving you the restoration and rejuvenation you need?

Track the quality of your sleep for one week by doing the following:

- Each day answer the nine questions on page 217 of *Dr. A's Habits of Health.*
- Use the Sleep Log in Appendix C (also available at www.habitsofhealth.net) to record your sleep. The sample Sleep Log will help you get started. Begin by recording the time you get into bed, the time you fall asleep, and the time you wake up.
- As the week goes on, you may start to see patterns emerge. Pay particular attention to any variation in your sleep schedule from work week to weekend. Does your sleep quality differ significantly?

PART THREE: EVALUATE YOUR SLEEP QUALITY

Answering the following questions will help you understand where you need to pay attention to your sleep quality.

When are you lacking sleep? _____

Do you nap? _____

Do you have a hard time getting up in the morning? _____

Did you find out from keeping the Sleep Log that your daily routine adversely affects your sleep? For example, are you drinking caffeine too late or drinking alcohol to "rest" your mind?

_____

On a scale of 1–10 (10 being perfect) evaluate the quality and quantity of your sleep:

_____

LIST YOUR PROBLEM AREAS.

_____

_____

_____

_____

_____

_____

PART FOUR: IMPROVE YOUR SLEEP QUALITY

Re-read step 3 on pages 218–220 of *Dr. A's Habits of Health*.

WRITE DOWN ANY IMMEDIATE CHANGES YOU'RE GOING TO MAKE IN YOUR DAILY ROUTINE TO IMPROVE THE QUALITY OF YOUR SLEEP.

_____

_____

_____

_____

_____

_____

> Sleep is the golden chain that ties health and our bodies together.
>
> — THOMAS DECKER, 1608

PART FIVE: IMPROVE YOUR BEDTIME ROUTINE AND ENVIRONMENT

It's important to create an environment that's conducive to sleep. Take a good look at yours, and then review the tips on creating an environment for sleep on page 221 of *Dr. A's Habits of Health*.

Is your bedroom soothing and inviting?_____

Does it relax you or stimulate you? _____

Is your bed comfortable? Does it support your body effectively? _____

Is the room or bed too hot or too cold? _____

YOUR STRUCTURAL TENSION CHART FOR HEALTHY SLEEP

Healthy Sleep:

Quality _____

Hours _____ Timeline

Secondary Choices

1. _____
2. _____
3. _____
4. _____
5. _____
6. _____
7. _____
8. _____
9. _____

_____

_____

_____

_____

_____

_____

_____

_____

_____

Quality _____

Hours _____

Current Reality

LESSON 14 ▶ Habits of Help and Helping

Create your own infrastructure of support to ensure a lifetime of success

BEFORE YOU BEGIN
Read Chapter 18 in *Dr. A's Habits of Health*

GOALS
- Understand the importance of support
- Identify potential healthy role models
- Share the Habits of Health with others
- Evaluate other potential areas of support
- Implement a daily support structure
- Create a structural tension chart for support

Research shows that people who seek support from others as they establish and reinforce positive life changes are more likely to succeed long term. As you move forward in your newly created world of healthy eating, motion, and sleep, relying on friends, family, co-workers, or a health coach can help you remain accountable for your actions—or lack thereof.

Building a support structure begins by identifying healthy role models. By this, I don't mean celebrities, athletes, or others you don't have a real relationship with, but rather friends, colleagues, relatives, and other people you know who are practicing the behaviors that you want in your life.

NAME FIVE PEOPLE YOU KNOW WHO ARE ACTIVELY WORKING TOWARD OPTIMAL HEALTH IN THEIR OWN LIVES.

1. _____
2. _____
3. _____
4. _____
5. _____

THE FULFILLMENT CONTINUUM

Your level of fulfillment is an internal measure of how you feel in your very being. Are you joyful, is your life full of meaning, or are you just plowing through the days like a hamster on a wheel? Re-read pages 267–272 in *Dr. A's Habits of Health* and mark your current position on the fulfillment continuum on the next page with a star.

Now mark where you were one year ago with a circle, and draw an arrow from that point to your current position. This will give you an objective idea of your current path. If you keep doing the same things you're doing now, where you will be in one, three, and five years from now?

Remember, just like your health you can change your direction if it's not in your favor. In fact, recognition is the first step.

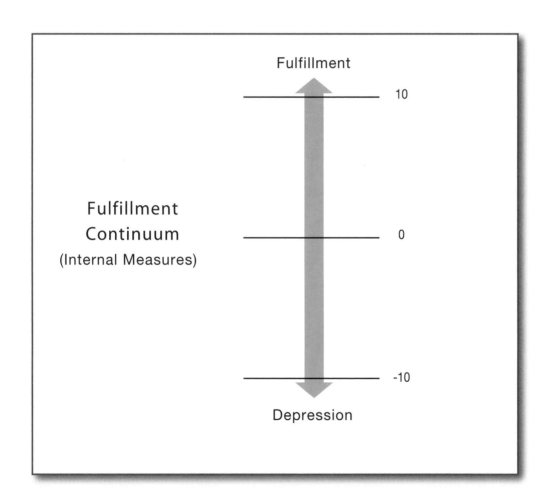

Create a structural tension chart to set that new direction. Spend some time writing down what you want to become, and what would bring you joy, a sense of being. A good way to begin is by saying, "I want to be…" *I want to be healthy. I want to be at peace with myself.* I want to be a house doesn't work, does it?

I WANT TO BE . . .

Your secondary choices are the things you're going to do to get there.

I'M GOING TO CREATE FULFILLMENT BY . . .

Fulfillment:

_____

_____

_____

Secondary Choices

1. _____
2. _____
3. _____
4. _____
5. _____
6. _____
7. _____
8. _____
9. _____

Timeline

_____

_____

_____

_____

_____

_____

_____

_____

_____

_____

_____

_____

Current Reality

THE SUCCESS CONTINUUM

Success is an external measure of what you have in terms of material things such as your career, home, or lifestyle. Although these things can't bring long-term joy and fulfillment, there's nothing wrong with striving to bring them into your world. Re-read pages 267–272 in *Dr. A's Habits of Health* and mark your current position on the success continuum below with a star.

Now mark where you were one year ago with a circle, and draw an arrow from that point to your current position. This will give you an objective idea of your current path. If you keep doing the same things you're doing now, where you will be in one, three, and five years from now?

As in the fulfillment chart, you can change your direction if it's not where you want to go.

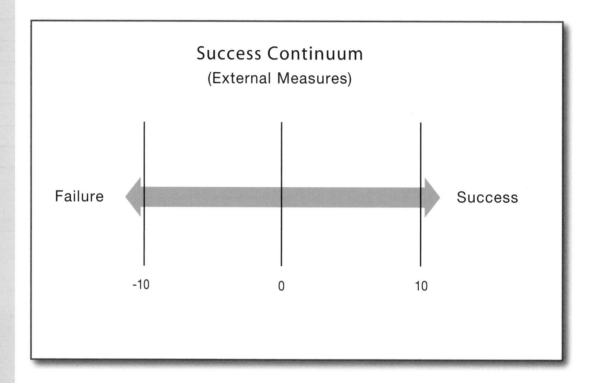

Create a structural tension chart to set that new direction. Spend some time writing down the things you want to have in your life—perhaps a new position at work or a new job altogether, a car, a house, a vacation, financial freedom…

I WANT TO HAVE . . .

_____

_____

_____

_____

_____

_____

_____

_____

Your secondary choices are the things you're going to do to get there.

I'M GOING TO CREATE SUCCESS BY . . .

_____

_____

_____

_____

_____

_____

_____

_____

_____

YOUR WELL-BEING CHART

On the well-being chart below, use both axes to mark your current position and where you want to be in terms of fulfillment and success. That's your direction and your focus, and puts you in the best possible position to thrive.

You may not get all of these things immediately, but what's more motivating and exciting than the possibility of guiding your life by what you want rather than what's thrown on you? And as a physician, I can tell you that if you're thriving you're much more likely to create optimal health.

Life is good! And I can tell you, it beats the heck out of just wearing the t-shirt!

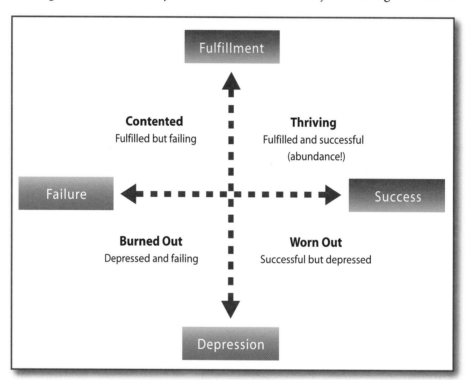

Most of us are used to setting and reaching goals for external objects such as a nice house or car, but it's important to ask yourself *why* you want what you want. Take another look at page 272 in *Dr. A's Habits of Health* for a more in-depth examination of this question.

It's also important that well-being and a love of life encompass a variety of experiences, gatherings, and people. Here are some ideas on ways to enrich your life right now. Describe how you might go about each one.

FOLLOW YOUR PASSION

TAKE UP A NEW HOBBY

ENJOY THE ARTS

EXPLORE NATURE

DEEPEN YOUR SPIRITUALITY OR SPEND MORE TIME WITH YOUR FAITH

WORK TOWARD A GOOD CAUSE OR WITH A CHARITY

SPEND TIME WITH OTHERS

_____

_____

_____

_____

Just remember to do what you love and love what you do…

This wonderful quote, which I keep over my desk, pretty much says it all:

The master in the art of living makes little distinction between his work and his play, his labor and his leisure, his mind and his body, his information and his recreation, his love and his religion. He hardly knows which is which. He simply pursues his vision of excellence at whatever he does, leaving others to decide whether he is working or playing. To him he's always doing both!

— JAMES A. MICHENER

For additional sources for creating well-being, see the resource list on page 370 of Dr. A's Habits of Health *and in the back of this workbook.*

LESSON 18 ▸ Habits of Longevity

Increase your longevity potential as you continue to improve your Habits of Health

BEFORE YOU BEGIN
Read Chapters 22 and 23 in *Dr. A's Habits of Health*

GOALS
- Learn about our normal lifespan
- Find out which factors determine aging
- Discover how and why people live into their 100s
- Apply habits that can help you live longer right now
- Create a structural tension chart for longevity

Having come this far, you're well equipped to be optimally healthy—as healthy as you can be with all that you are. Doesn't it make sense now to take the next step and seize the potential for a longer life?

Without the Habits of Health, your chances of living longer are really just wishful thinking. But with them, you've gained control of your energy management system. Now we're going to help you squeeze out more healthy years by refining that system even further.

PRINCIPLES OF LONGEVITY

Let's start with some questions on the principles of longevity, based on Chapter 22 in *Dr. A's Habits of Health.*

(HOH page 279)
What's the first principle of longevity? _____

Is aging reversible? _____

Improving life expectancy starts within _____ months of starting the Habits of Health.

What percentage do your genes play in your longevity? _____

What percentage do your lifestyle and behaviors play? _____

(HOH page 280)
How long does the average woman live?_____ The average man?_____

What do biological and chronological age mean? _____

_____

_____

_____

What two cellular structures may determine our aging? _____

Name two things that may keep these structures healthy. _____

_____

(HOH page 282)
What may be our best bet for a longer life? _____

Some of the most important work on longevity has been through studies of groups of people who have actually lived to be over 100. The Okinawans, Sardinians, and U.S. centenarians have habits that have been attributed to their longevity. **NAME FIVE OF THESE HABITS.** (HOH pages 286–287)

1. _____

2. _____

3. _____

4. _____

5. _____

As we unravel the secrets of aging in our genes, there's one thing that's absolutely certain—that if applied consistently, a lifestyle based on _____ can help extend your life!

HABITS OF LONGEVITY

Let's find out more about longevity and lifespan by answering some questions based on Chapter 23 of *Dr. A's Habits of Health*.

(HOH pages 290–291)
What are the two principles of aging?

1. _____

2. _____

What is the average human life expectancy? _____

What is the actual maximum human lifespan? _____

What is the predicted maximum? _____

What is the principle of secondary aging? _____

_____

_____

_____

The insidious decay in our organ systems is the direct result of our obesigenic world and our Habits of Disease. Our medical delivery system is poised to respond to this decay, but much like trying to salvage a badly rusting car, it may slow down the process but never return the car (or your unhealthy body) back to showroom quality. For that, you need the Habits of Health—and they need to be applied fully.

What is the key organ affected by secondary aging? _____

(In fact, this particular organ is so important that we're going to spend the whole of lesson 20 addressing its optimization!)

DR. A'S LONGEVITY PLAN

There are a number of things that you can change right now to reduce your likelihood of falling prey to preventable diseases, accidents, and the ravages of an unhealthy lifestyle. They're outlined on pages 293–296 of *Dr. A's Habits of Health*, but let's go over them again here.

Step 1: Right Now

CHECK OFF THE CHANGES YOU'VE MASTERED.

- ☐ Don't use tobacco
- ☐ Don't use recreational drugs
- ☐ Wear seatbelts
- ☐ Drive a car with airbags
- ☐ Drive the speed limit
- ☐ Limit alcohol
- ☐ Practice safe sex
- ☐ Avoid sunburn
- ☐ Avoid highways

139

Your first priority is to master any remaining unchecked risks. Review lessons 2 and 3 to learn how to harness them.

Step 2: Create a Healthy Environment

CHECK OFF THE CHANGES YOU'VE MASTERED.

- ☐ Eliminate toxins
- ☐ Purify your water
- ☐ Purify your air
- ☐ Equip your house with functioning smoke detectors
- ☐ Create swimming pool barriers
- ☐ Secure your home
- ☐ Secure firearms

Step 3: Get a Yearly Check-Up

Be sure to address all health issues with your physician and ask for their cooperation as you continue to adopt and strengthen your Habits of Health.

Let them know that you want to create optimal health and minimize the need for medications. (See page 294 of *Dr. A's Habits of Health*.) You might even want to share with them the story in Appendix E of this workbook, of the journey from traditional Western medicine to the third era of medicine, written by one of my new health professionals!

Step 4: Create Optimal Oral Health

CHECK OFF THE CHANGES YOU'VE MASTERED.

- ☐ Brush your teeth at least twice a day with fluoride toothpaste
- ☐ Floss daily
- ☐ Get a yearly dental check-up
- ☐ Have your teeth cleaned twice a year
- ☐ Don't use tobacco products
- ☐ Limit alcohol
- ☐ Use lip balm with sunscreen
- ☐ Avoid lipsticks without sunscreen
- ☐ Keep your mouth moist

Step 5: Reach and Maintain Your Healthy Weight

CHECK OFF THE CHANGES YOU'VE MASTERED.

- ☐ Habits of Healthy Eating
- ☐ BeSlim
- ☐ Habits of Motion

Step 6: Incorporate the Habits of Health

CHECK OFF THE CHANGES YOU'VE MASTERED.

- ☐ The three habits listed above
- ☐ Habits of healthy sleeping
- ☐ Optimum support
- ☐ Anti-inflammatory strategy
- ☐ Nutritional optimization and augmentation

Step 7: Attain Optimal Health

Dr. A's Habits of Health and this companion guide have given you a roadmap to create and sustain optimal health for now and for always. But it's your responsibility to progressively implement all of this material in order to enjoy the full benefit of this program. Get some help, have some fun, apply structural tension, proper motivation, and primary and secondary choices—and enjoy a thriving life.

Give it time! This isn't a sprint, but an amazing journey to uncover your healthy vibrant self. Once you have a firm handle on the Habits of Health and they've become the thick cable we described in lesson 2, you'll be ready for the final frontier . . . if you choose it.

ULTRAHEALTH

This advanced program—designed to potentially help you live longer—isn't for everyone.

Although it incorporates the latest, cutting-edge scientific research, it's not a magic potion. Rather, it's a refinement that moves your body into a state of ultra-efficiency. And by its very nature, it will require choices that are driven by a dynamic urge to live longer. You'll eat less, eliminate processed food entirely, move at a more intense pace. If that sounds like a choice you want to take, then let's go for it!

First, have some fun and create a structural tension chart for your longevity. Now, no one can predict when our expiration date will really come, but if we have a strong, dynamic urge to live a longer, healthier life and make the secondary choices that support our vision, who knows what's possible?

Just so you know, my goal for a maximum optimal healthy age is 130. Move over, Jeanne Louise Calment!

YOUR STRUCTURAL TENSION CHART FOR MAXIMUM OPTIMALLY HEALTHY AGE

Maximum Optimally Healthy Age

_____ years old

Secondary Choices

1. Reach a healthy weight
2. Model the Habits of Health
3. Maintain optimal health for age
4. Adopt Dr. A's longevity plan
5. _____
6. _____
7. _____
8. _____
9. _____
10. _____
11. _____
12. _____
13. _____
14. _____
15. _____

Timeline

_____
_____
_____
_____
_____
_____
_____
_____
_____
_____
_____
_____

_____ years old

Current Reality

LESSON 19 ▶ Ultrahealth—Living Longer Full Out

Expand your Habits of Health
for a longer life

BEFORE YOU BEGIN
Read Chapter 24 in *Dr. A's Habits of Health*

GOALS
- Understand what determines your lifespan
- Discover what Ultrahealth looks like
- Create your Ultrahealth dietary optimization and movement enhancement plans
- Create a structural tension chart for reaching Ultrahealth

ULTRAHEALTH: THE FINAL STEP

As you learned in Chapter 24 of *Dr. A's Habits of Health*, your lifespan is determined by three factors.

WHAT ARE THOSE FACTORS AND HOW MUCH INFLUENCE DOES EACH ONE HAVE? (HOH page 296)

1. _____ _____ %
2. _____ _____ %
3. _____ _____ %

WHAT DOES ULTRAHEALTH LOOK LIKE?

When you reach Ultrahealth, your body functions in a state of maximum efficiency. You'll learn to thrive on fewer calories, less sugar, whole foods, and more intense, focused movement. As a result, your body will actually change its blood chemistry and lower its inflammatory state.

We're talking about a whole new standard for health optimization. Your lab results will compare with those of an Olympic-trained athlete. Your physician will be astonished; you'll be the healthiest person he'll have seen all day!

The key parameters include:

- Blood pressure readings in the 110–95 mmHg range (systolic) and 75–65 mmHg range (diastolic) (mmHg = millimeters of mercury, the units used to measure blood pressure)
- A BMI (body mass index) in the low 20s
- Body fat measurements as low as 10% for men and 17% for women
- An hs-CRP (a measurement of inflammation) below 0.5mg/L

It all adds up to a state of thriving that may just slow down your cellular aging!

So if this is your primary choice, let's talk about the secondary choices that will bring it into being.

DR. A'S ULTRAHEALTH PLAN

LIST THE THREE MAJOR FOCUS AREAS FOR ULTRAHEALTH. (HOH page 298)

1. _____
2. _____
3. _____

In this lesson, we'll focus on the first two areas of my Ultrahealth program:

- Dietary optimization
- Movement enhancement

And in the next lesson, we'll turn our attention to brain health optimization and preservation.

DIETARY OPTIMIZATION

In the three phases of energy management that you learned about in *Dr. A's Habits of Health* (see diagram, page 277), we focused on creating a very tight balance of energy in and energy out.

In phase I, we helped you reach a healthy weight by lowering your energy intake to facilitate your use of your unhealthy belly fat as an energy source. In phase II, we equilibrated your energy in and out as you learned how to eat a full range of healthy foods for life. Phase III was a tight optimization to match energy in and out as you started changing your body composition by adding muscle and decreased your percentage of body fat.

In phase IV, we're going to create a state of Ultrahealth by lowering your total daily caloric intake compared to what's considered the norm. Now, the calorie restriction groups I discuss in *Dr. A's Habits of Health* drop their caloric intake by 30%, but that isn't sustainable for most people. So instead, we're going to cut your calories by just 15% and drop the other 15% by increasing your energy expenditure. This decrease in calories will be offset by the fact that your dietary intake will be made up primarily of nutrient-dense food.

QUALIFICATIONS FOR THE ULTRAHEALTH PROGRAM

To take part in the Ultrahealth program, the following are required:

- ☐ A state of optimal health for at least six months (preferably a year)
- ☐ Healthy weight for at least six months (preferably a year)
- ☐ Normal lab work (see page 299 in *Dr. A's Habits of Health*)
- ☐ Approval by your primary care physician
- ☐ A visit to your primary care physician every three months for the first year

Warning! Do not allow your BMI to fall below 20. Monitor your progress closely under the direct supervision of your physician. Anyone with a history of eating disorders, immune suppression, or other wasting disorders should not use this program.

Note: If you don't fit these criteria, or just don't feel you're ready yet, you can skip ahead to the next lesson, which focuses on brain longevity.

ULTRAHEALTH REQUIREMENTS

Part One: Ultrahealth Daily Caloric Intake
We'll start by recalculating your new Ultrahealth daily caloric intake, using our old friend Total Energy Expenditure (TEE) (see page 300 in *Dr. A's Habits of Health*.)

Step 1: Basal metabolic rate (BMR)
Now that you've reached optimal health, we'll use the more accurate equation to calculate your BMR:

Male:
BMR = 10 x (your weight in pounds x 0.455) x (height in inches) - 5 x (age) + 5: _____

Female:

BMR = 10 x (your weight in pounds x 0.455) x (height in inches) - 5 x (age) - 161: _____

Step 2: Physical activity level (PAL)

Now use your BMR from the equation above and take into account your activity level, using the Activity Factor Table on page 156 of *Dr. A's Habits of Health*. This modified BMR is called your EEpal.

EEpal = BMR x activity factor: _____

Step 3: Thermic effect of food (TEF)

This calculation takes into account the calories that are required to process your food. It averages around 10%.

TEF = EEpal x 0.1: _____

Step 4: Optimal health TEE

This is calculated by adding your TEF to your EEpal.

Optimal health TEE = EEpal + TEF: _____

Step 5: Calculate your Ultrahealth daily energy intake

Now calculate 85% of your optimal health TEE, above. This figure is your Ultrahealth daily energy intake (UDEA), and represents a 15% reduction in calories from your optimal health level. (Remember, we want this to be sustainable.)

Ultrahealth daily energy intake (UDEI) = optimal health TEE x 0.85: _____

This number is your new goal for daily calorie intake.

Part Two: Ultrahealth Daily Food Intake

Now we're going to optimize your diet by shifting away from energy-dense, nutritionally deficient food to a new regimen of energy-sparse, nutrient-dense food. You've already incorporated many of these foods into your diet as you moved toward optimal health. We're simply going to eliminate any foods that can spur inflammation and insulin production.

To do that, you're going to eliminate processed food and eat only nutrient-filled, low-glycemic carbohydrates, lean protein, and healthy fats. Here's how your new diet will look:

- Reduced daily caloric intake
- No processed food
- Lowest-glycemic carbohydrates
- Increased soy intake (based on Okinawan longevity studies)
- Healthy fats, especially olive oil, fish, walnuts, and flaxseed
- Eating every three hours

You'll find a sample Ultrahealth daily meal plan on page 301 of *Dr. A's Habits of Health*. You should also be supplementing with all the required vitanutrients that apply to you, as discussed in lesson 16.

Now let's focus on how we're going to reach the other 15% energy adjustment from my enhanced movement plan.

Part Three: Ultrahealth Exercise Enhancement

To increase your energy expenditure, you're going to add more movement to your weekly routine. You'll find that this addition will fit very nicely into your current movement plan and won't really take up much more time.

First, take the optimal health TEE that you calculated above.

Optimal health TEE x 0.15 = additional energy expenditure in kcal twice a week

We're going to add this to your very active NEAT and EAT System programs to increase your average daily energy expenditure by 15% over your optimal health TEE. You'll burn this additional 150–500 calories by intensifying your workouts.

To do this, you'll start by adding two additional activities to your current EAT System program. You can choose either the EAT resistance or EAT walking program, based on where you feel you're more accomplished.

Beginning on page 303 of *Dr. A's Habits of Health*, you'll find six options for boosting your EAT resistance workouts and two options (interval A or B) for intensifying your EAT walking program. Choose one of these to add to your existing schedule twice a week until it becomes routine. You can then change your resistance or walking option, or mix it up and do one resistance option and one walking enhancement.

Review the sample weekly Ultrahealth movement plan on page 305 of *Dr. A's Habits of Health*. Then determine your own plan by filling out the blank movement plan in Appendix F of this workbook (also available at www.habitsofhealth.net).

WHAT ARE THE FOUR COMPONENTS OF YOUR ULTRAHEALTH MOVEMENT PLAN?
(HOH page 306)

1. _____

2. _____

3. _____

4. _____

Below you'll find a structural tension chart for achieving Ultrahealth.

YOUR STRUCTURAL TENSION CHART FOR REACHING ULTRAHEALTH

Ultrahealth Lifestyle:
Dietary Optimization
Movement Enhancement
Brain Optimization

Secondary Choices

1. Reduced daily calories 15%
2. Added 15% increase in EE
3. Brain exercises daily
4. Brain food intake daily
5. _____
6. _____
7. _____
8. _____
9. _____

Timeline

_____
_____
_____
_____
_____
_____
_____
_____
_____
_____
_____

Optimal Health > 6 months

Current Reality

You now have a solid dietary optimization and movement plan to improve your cellular health and potentially live a longer life. Now let's turn our attention to the master controller of aging—your brain.

LESSON 20 ▸ Keeping Your Healthy Brain

Keep your CPU in top condition, sharpen your memory, and extend your life

BEFORE YOU BEGIN
Read Chapter 25 in *Dr. A's Habits of Health*

GOALS
- Learn what's needed to keep your brain healthy and functioning well
- Choose new habits that will enhance your brain for life
- Understand the role of exercise in keeping your brain healthy
- Understand the role of proper nutrition on brain function
- Create a structural tension chart for brain optimization

Is your brain working or on vacation?

To live longer in a healthy state, learning how to optimize and protect your brain is paramount. Most of us take for granted that our brain is "good to go" and doesn't need tending to, but as you learned in Chapter 25 of *Dr. A's Habits of Health,* that's just not so!

Let's review the specific habits that will protect and enhance your brain and enable it to continue directing you toward a state of ever-increasing health.

LIST THE THREE MAJOR AREAS ESSENTIAL FOR BRAIN HEALTH AND LONGEVITY. (HOH page 307)

1. _____

2. _____

3. _____

YOUR BRAIN WILL PROVIDE OPTIMAL LEVELS OF COGNITION AND MEMORY AS LONG AS YOU MAINTAIN IT UNDER THESE IMPORTANT CONDITIONS. (HOH page 307)

1. _____

2. _____

3. _____

Re-read the section on neurons on page 308 of *Dr. A's Habits of Health*, and you'll gain a greater appreciation for the abilities of your brain. Based on 100 billion neurons with 10,000 synapses each, that's a total of _____ connections. Amazing!

As you've learned, our brains need a workout just as much as our bodies do.

LIST SOME ACTIVITIES YOU CAN DO TO EXERCISE YOUR BRAIN. (HOH page 309)

1. _____

2. _____

3. _____

4. _____

5. _____

WHAT EVERYDAY TASKS CAN YOU SWITCH AROUND (by shutting your eyes or using your non-dominant hand, for example) to create new neural pathways? (HOH page 309)

1. _____

2. _____

3. _____

4. _____

LIST THE MENTAL PRACTICES THAT WILL BOOST YOUR BRAIN'S ABILITY TO LEARN.
(HOH page 310)

1. _____
2. _____
3. _____
4. _____
5. _____
6. _____

PHYSICAL EXERCISE AND THE BRAIN

Adults who exercise at least three days a week have a substantially lower risk of developing dementia later in life compared with those who don't exercise.

WHY IS PHYSICAL EXERCISE SO IMPORTANT FOR BRAIN FUNCTION? (HOH page 311)

1. _____
2. _____
3. _____

WHAT MAKES FOR A HEALTHY BRAIN ENVIRONMENT? (HOH page 311)

_____
_____

Nerve Growth Factor (NGF) is produced in the brain and stimulated by exercise.

WHAT DOES NGF DO, AND WHY IS IT IMPORTANT? (HOH page 312)

_____
_____

Physical exercise has been shown to reduce stress, which in turn helps keep the brain free of damaging substances that create dysfunction.

WHAT ARE SOME OTHER PRACTICES YOU CAN ADOPT TO REDUCE STRESS?
(HOH pages 313–315)

1. _____
2. _____
3. _____
4. _____
5. _____

FEED YOUR HEAD!

Certain foods and supplements are particularly important for brain health and longevity.

WHY IS YOUR BRAIN ESPECIALLY VULNERABLE TO ATTACK BY DESTRUCTIVE OXYGEN RADICALS? (HOH page 316)

_____
_____

WHICH FATS ARE IMPORTANT TO AVOID? (HOH page 316)

_____
_____

WHICH FATS CAN YOU ENJOY? (HOH page 316)

1. _____
2. _____
3. _____
4. _____

The best carbohydrates to choose are those that are _____ glycemic. (HOH page 316)

On page 317 of *Dr. A's Habits of Health*, you'll find a great list of supplements for brain health.

WHICH SUPPLEMENTS WILL YOU ADD TO YOUR DAILY REGIMEN?

1. _____
2. _____
3. _____
4. _____
5. _____

I hope you now have a better appreciation of how well the brain responds to exercise and nutrition. It really makes it easy for us to take care of our most precious organ!

YOUR STRUCTURAL TENSION CHART FOR BRAIN OPTIMIZATION

Brain Optimization:

_____

_____

Secondary Choices

1. Brain exercises

2. _____

3. _____

4. _____

5. Stress reduction techniques

6. _____

7. _____

8. _____

9. Brain foods

10. _____

11. _____

12. _____

Timeline

_____

_____

_____

_____

_____

_____

_____

_____

_____

_____

_____

_____

_____

_____

Current Reality

LESSON 21 ▸ Lessons of Ultrahealth

What's next? Discover cutting-edge scientific research that can help you thrive into your eighties, nineties, and beyond

BEFORE YOU BEGIN
Read Chapter 26 in *Dr. A's Habits of Health*

GOALS

- Learn the goals of Ultrahealth
- Set your time schedule for reaching Ultrahealth
- Review the potential benefits of resveratrol
- Understand why Ultrahealth is currently your best chance for longevity
- Create a structural tension chart for reaching Ultrahealth

As you begin your Ultrahealth program, it's extremely important to monitor your progress. Although we're really only expanding your optimal health program to a higher level, and we anticipate that your body is going to thrive, we still want to be cautious, especially if you've had health issues or have been on medications.

Be sure to see your physician after your first month on the Ultrahealth plan, or sooner if needed.

YOUR PHYSICIAN WILL PROBABLY OBSERVE THESE OUTSTANDING HEALTH OUTCOMES.
(HOH page 318)

1. _____
2. _____
3. _____
4. _____

GOALS OF ULTRAHEALTH

There are three key parameters we'll use to guide your progress and actually define the point when you begin experiencing an Ultrahealth state.

WHAT ARE THESE PARAMETERS? (HOH page 318)

1. _____

2. _____

3. _____

1. High-sensitivity C-reactive protein (hs-CRP)

You may need to ask your doctor for the high-sensitivity (hs) version of this test, which is not normally done. I love this marker because it gives you a great indication of the health of your *whole* body.

What are the CDC's criteria for disease risk based on hs-CRP? (HOH page 319)

Low risk _____ mg/l

Average risk _____ mg/l

High risk _____ mg/l

Our first goal is to lower your hs-CRP to less than _____ mg/l. (HOH page 319)

Our Ultrahealth goal will be a steady state of less than _____ mg/l. (HOH page 319)

2. Body mass index (BMI)

Your body mass index is an easy measurement you can use to track your progress. Just as before, when we lowered it to less than 25 in order to lower your risk of disease, it must be taken in context with your waist circumference, because visceral adiposity (the fat around your middle) is the most critical fat to eliminate.

In a state of optimal health, a healthy BMI is under 25, with a waist circumference of less than 35 inches for men and less than 31 inches for women.

For Ultrahealth, you'll want to reach a BMI in the low 20s—but more importantly a waist circumference of less than 32 inches for men and less than 29 inches for women. (The exact number will vary somewhat for different body types.)

3. Body fat percentage

Optimal body fat percentage varies according to genetics, culture, and environment, but for a good guideline, see the chart on page 320 of *Dr. A's Habits of Health.*

WHY IS IT HEALTHY FOR WOMEN TO HAVE A HIGHER PERCENTAGE OF BODY FAT?
(HOH page 320)

_____

_____

_____

If you're a woman, your body fat percentage goal is _____. (HOH page 320)

If you're a man, your body fat percentage goals is _____. (HOH page 320)

CALORIE RESTRICTION

Calorie restriction is a natural extension of the Habits of Health energy management system that's at the core of our program and has helped you take control of your health.

When combined with a rich low-glycemic, nutrient-dense diet and the elimination of processed food, there's good reason to believe that this strategy will work to extend life in humans. It's already been shown to be successful in animals, including some encouraging early data in primates.

I'm convinced that, at the very least, this combination will have a positive impact on disease reduction and quality of health and life in those who subscribe to Ultrahealth.

WINE: HEALTH BENEFITS AND LONGEVITY

Wine has drawn significant interest in longevity research. We're not yet sure whether wine is the answer to living longer, but it's an intriguing question.

Red wine stands out as the gold standard, based on its heavy concentration of over 200 different substances that have antioxidant properties. These phenolic compounds may indeed contribute to the growing body of research on the health benefits of wine.

Even more exciting, recent research has uncovered a compound in red wine that seems to increase the lifespan of animals, much like the benefits of calorie restriction.

That compound is called _____ . (HOH page 322)

It's also been discovered that this polyphenolic compound exists in higher quantities in red wines that are grown in hostile environments, such as higher elevations that receive more ultra-violet rays, and in cool, damp environments.

WHAT ARE SOME OF THE HEALTH BENEFITS OF RESVERATROL? (HOH page 322)

1. _____
2. _____
3. _____
4. _____
5. _____

WHICH WINES HAVE THE HIGHEST CONCENTRATION OF RESVERATROL? (HOH page 323)

1. _____
2. _____
3. _____

SHOULD I DRINK RED WINE? (HOH page 323)

If I don't currently drink: yes _____   no _____

If I do currently drink: yes _____   no _____   maybe _____

We still don't know whether consuming wine *in moderation*—specifically red wine—is a good strategy for health and longevity. Right now, there's no strong reason to start or stop drinking it. Whatever your decision, make sure it's in line with the secondary choices that support your foundations of health. If you're still struggling with your calorie intake and resulting weight gain, it probably makes sense to stop. If you already drink some other form of alcohol and don't intend to quit, then converting to red wine in moderation makes sense.

But please drink responsibly! (See information regarding alcohol consumption on page 324 of *Dr. A's Habits of Health*.)

ON THE HORIZON: SENSE AND SCIENCE

In our lifetime, science has changed the landscape of our world. It has put us as physicians in position to make significant headway in our war on disease.

The global scientific community and the Internet have enabled us to unravel the code of DNA, and with those findings create treatments for previously incurable diseases. We're learning what causes our cells and bodies to age at an accelerative pace. And with the advance of nanotechnology (a science that enables us to insert miniaturized materials into our bodies), it's just a matter of time before we have the capability to extend life.

Yet if you look at the U.S. today, you can see that our longer life expectancy—the longest in human history—has come at a great cost. Technology is capable of extending our life, but at the same time it's filled us with cheap, nutritionally polluted, high-calorie processed foods and robbed us of adequate movement.

Using technology to react to symptoms caused by the Habits of Disease lifestyle is no longer affordable or desirable. And the same is true of our focus on prolonging life through technological means. Does it make sense to use technology to keep unhealthy people alive longer at great expense and great suffering?

This leads me to our final exercise. In lesson 2, you answered yes to the question, "If you had a choice to live in optimal health, would you take it?"

The question I have for you now is this:

If learning and implementing the Habits of Health can put you on track to create optimal health, move toward Ultrahealth, and potentially live a longer, healthier life—are you willing to adopt the secondary daily choices to support that goal?

If your answer is yes, I have some very good news for you. The longevity breakthroughs of the future will fully benefit only one group—those who are optimally healthy.

Congratulations, and enjoy!

YOUR STRUCTURAL TENSION CHART
FOR REACHING ULTRAHEALTH

Ultrahealth State:

Hs-CRP < .5 mg/l

BMI 20-24

Body Fat F 17% M 10%

Secondary Choices

1. Reduced daily calories 15%
2. Added 15% increase in EE
3. Brain exercises daily
4. Brain food intake daily
5. _____
6. _____
7. _____
8. _____

Timeline

_____
_____
_____
_____
_____
_____
_____
_____

Hs-CRP _____ mg/l

BMI _____

Body Fat _____

Current Reality

APPENDIX A

Physician Information

Your patient has made the fundamental choice to create health in his or her life by taking part in a comprehensive health-modification program, the first step of which is reaching a healthy weight.

I've asked them to share this information with you to ensure that they have the proper medical supervision as they undergo this transformation to optimal health. The following is a brief description of the program and some suggested medical support.

- **Phase I: Weight Loss**
  ✓ Calorie reduction
  ✓ Dietary focus on low-glycemic carbohydrates, healthy fats, and proteins
  ✓ q. 3-hour portion control using medically formulated, low-calorie, portion-controlled meal replacements (PCMRs)
  ✓ Instruction in healthy eating system
  ✓ Increased daily movement

- **Phase II: Lifestyle Change**
  ✓ Healthy eating for life
  ✓ Increased exercise through daily walking plan and resistance training
  ✓ Improved sleeping patterns
  ✓ Support through personal coach, online tracking, and/or bionetwork health community
  ✓ Ongoing instruction through Habits of Health book and workbook
  ✓ Behavioral changes through focus on motivation and choices to support health

- **Phase III: Creating a Microenvironment of Health**
  ✓ Removal of inflammatory stimulators (i.e., water, air, and home toxins)
  ✓ Stress reduction
  ✓ Enhancement of healthy nutrients

Your patient will be eating a reduced amount of energy-dense, low-glycemic food and will lose two to five pounds per week for the first two weeks, 1–2 pounds per week thereafter. As a result, their blood sugar, cholesterol, triglycerides, blood pressure, and hs-CRP could possibly decrease. Diabetics should lower their hypoglycemic medications and increase blood sugar monitoring as they begin this new eating pattern to avoid hypoglycemia.

Suggested Diagnostics

In addition to routine blood chemistry, suggested labs include lipid profile for a baseline, hs-CRP, and EKG. A cardiovascular assessment is suggested in high-risk individuals especially if they have considerable weight to lose or have been inactive.

Significant Disease Caution

The presence of significant medical conditions and certain medications may prohibit or severely limit the use of this program. Because of the calorie restriction and speed of weight loss involved, the program is not recommended for patients with the following conditions: heart attack within the past three months; recent or recurrent strokes or mini-strokes; unstable angina; severe liver or kidney disease; clotting disorders; active cancers; eating disorders; severe psychiatric disturbances; current use of steroids over 20 mg/day; current use of lithium; or type 1 diabetes.

For more information on our program, go to www.habitsofhealth.net or contact a health coach.

APPENDIX B

Note: The charts in Appendix B can be downloaded from the Web site at www.habitsofhealth.net.

NEAT Scoring Sheet

Category	NEAT Points	Energy Expenditure
Stance (Posture)		
Core position focus	1 point per minute	1 kcal/min
Balance ball	10 points per hour	10 kcal/hour
Sitting to moving	1 point	1 kcal
Standing		
Standing upright	1 point per minute	1 kcal/min

Strolling (Walking)

1. Record your total steps per day (TSD).
2. Divide your TSD by your Energetic Step Value ESV (see chart) to find your NEAT points.

ENERGETIC STEP VALUE (ESV)
(steps required to burn 1 kcal)

Body Mass Index BMI	ESV (Female)	ESV (Male)
18 – 24.9 Healthy	36 steps per kcal	28 steps per kcal
25 – 29.9 Overweight	30 steps per kcal	24 steps per kcal
30 – 34.9 Class I Obesity	24 steps per kcal	20 steps per kcal
35 – 39.9 Class II Obesity	18 steps per kcal	16 steps per kcal
Over 40 Class III Obesity	12 steps per kcal	11 steps per kcal

Energetic Step Value (ESV) (steps required to burn 1 kcal). Locate your BMI in the left-hand column of the chart to find out how many steps you must take to burn one calorie. This number is your Energetic Step Value (ESV), which you'll use to calculate the total number of NEAT points you earn from walking.

Stairs

1. Record the flights of stairs you climb (up and down) per day.
2. Multiply that number by your NEAT points per flight (see chart) to find your total NEAT points.

NEAT Points per Flight of Stairs. Locate your BMI in the left-hand column to find out how many NEAT points you earn for each flight of stairs you climb.

NEAT POINTS PER FLIGHT OF STAIRS	
Body Mass Index BMI	NEAT Points per flight (up and down)
<25	3
25 – 30	4
30 – 35	5
35 – 40	6
>40	7

Samba

Listening to music (up-tempo)	1 point per minute	1 kcal/min
Slow to moderate dancing	3 points per minute	3 kcal/min
Fast to intense dancing	5 points per minute	5 kcal/min

Switch

Minor manual task	1 point per task	1 kcal
Manual chore	3 points per minute	3 kcal/min

Daily NEAT Activity Log

	Stance	Standing	Strolling	Stairs	Samba	Switch
7:00 – 8:00 am						
8:00 – 9:00 am						
9:00 – 10:00 am						
10:00 – 11:00 am						
11:00 – 12:00 am						
12:00 – 1:00 pm						
1:00 – 2:00 pm						
2:00 – 3:00 pm						
3:00 – 4:00 pm						
4:00 – 5:00 pm						
5:00 – 6:00 pm						
6:00 – 7:00 pm						
7:00 – 8:00 pm						
8:00 – 9:00 pm						
9:00 – 10:00 pm						
Total						
	Core position (minutes) _____ Balance ball (hours) _____ Sitting to moving _____	Minutes _____	Total steps per day (TSD) _____ Energetic Step Value _____	Flights per day _____ NEAT points per flight _____	Music (minutes) _____ Slow dance (minutes) _____ Fast dance (minutes) _____	Tasks _____ Chores (minutes) _____
NEAT Points						
NEAT Point Guide	Core position focus 1 point per minute Balance ball 10 points per hour Sitting to moving 1 point	Standing 1 point per minute	TSD ÷ ESV = total NEAT points	Flights (up and down) x points per flight = total NEAT points	Upbeat music 1 point per minute Slow dance 3 points per minute Fast dance 5 points per minute	Manual task 1 point Manual chore 3 points per minute

Weekly NEAT Activity Log

NEAT Points	Monday	Tuesday	Wednesday	Thursday	Friday	Saturday	Sunday	Total NEAT Points
Stance								
Standing								
Strolling								
Stairs								
Samba								
Switch								

NEAT Goal Setter

Your goals for this initial stage of your lifetime movement plan are as follows:

- 120 NEAT points per day for the first thirty days.
- 200 NEAT points per day for the second thirty days.

	ADD 1 NEW NEAT "S" ACTIVITY PER DAY
DAY 1	
DAY 2	
DAY 3	
DAY 4	
DAY 5	
DAY 6	
DAY 7	

Depending on your current lifestyle and activity level, I suggest you focus on adding one additional activity per day for the first week, then one additional activity in each category starting the second week, until you've reached 200 NEAT points per day.

Starting in the second week, add one additional NEAT "S" activity per week in each category.

	S	+ S	+ S	+ S	+ S	+ S
WEEK 2 Add 1 activity per category						
WEEK 3 Add 1 activity per category						
WEEK 4 Add 1 activity per category						

APPENDIX C

Note: The charts in Appendix C can be downloaded from the Web site at www.habitsofhealth.net.

Rate of Perceived Exertion (Borg Scale)

Adapted from Borg, G. V., "Psychological Basis of Perceived Exertion," *Medicine and Science Sports* 14 (1982): 377–81.

EAT Walking Program Daily Tracking Sheet

RATE OF PERCEIVED EXERTION

Borg Scale	RPE
0	nothing at all
0.5	very, very light
1	very light
2	light
3	moderate
4	somewhat hard
5 – 6	hard
7 – 8	very hard
9	very, very hard
10	maximum exertion

Day	Warm-Up	Time	Cool-Down	Steps	Miles*	Calories
Day 1						
Day 2						
Day 3						
Day 4						
Day 5						
Day 6						
Day 7						
Day 8						
Day 9						
Day 10						
Day 11						
Day 12						
Day 13						
Day 14						

*1 mile = 2,000 steps

EAT Walking Program Weekly Tracking Sheet

Week	Steps per Day		Steps per Week	Miles*	Comments
	Actual	Recommended			
1		1,000/day			
2		1,200/day			
3		1,400/day			
4		1,600/day			
5		1,800/day			
6		2,000/day			
7		2,500/day			
8		3,000/day			
9		3,500/day			
10		4,000/day			
11		4,500/day			
12		5,000/day			
13		5,500/day			
14		6,000/day			

*1 mile = 2,000 steps

EAT Resistance Program Training Log: Upper Body

Muscle Group	Exercise / Level (level one, level two)	Weight: Body (B) or Pounds (lbs)	Rate of Perceived Exertion (RPE)
Rotation A			
Core			
Chest			
Back			
Shoulders			
Arms			
Rotation B			
Core			
Chest			
Back			
Shoulders			
Arms			

EAT Resistance Program Training Log: Lower Body

Muscle Group	Exercise / Level (level one, level two)	Weight: Body (B) or Pounds (lbs)	Rate of Perceived Exertion (RPE)
Rotation A			
Core			
Thighs			
Gluteals			
Hamstrings			
Calves			
Rotation B			
Core			
Thighs			
Gluteals			
Hamstrings			
Calves			

APPENDIX D

Note: The charts in Appendix D can be downloaded from the Web site at www.habitsofhealth.net.

Sleep Log

The Sleep Log is designed to help you figure out which behaviors are affecting your sleep. To use the log:

- Answer the following questions, from part two of the sleep assessment on page 217 of *Dr. A's Habits of Health,* every day for one week.
- Each day, enter your answers in the log on page 167, using the symbols in the key.

1. What time did you get into bed last night?

2. What time did you get out of bed in the morning?

3. What hours did you actually sleep?

4. Did you take a nap? For how long?

5. Did you consume alcohol? How much, and at what time?

6. Did you exercise? How long, and at what time?

7. Did you drink coffee or other caffeinated beverages? How much, and at what time?

8. What hours did you watch television?

9. Did you take any medications? At what time?

To help you get started, take a look at the sample sleep log on the next page.

Sample Sleep Log

TIME	SUN–MON	MON–TUES	TUES–WED	WED–THURS	THURS–FRI	FRI–SAT	SAT–SUN
6:00 PM				E			
7:00 PM	TV					A	
8:00 PM		TV	C		A	A	
9:00 PM		TV	TV				
10:00 PM	F	○	TV	TV	A	A, F	
11:00 PM	○		○	TV	A	A, F	
MIDNIGHT				○			○
1:00 AM	●	●	●		○●	○●	
2:00 AM				●	●	●	
3:00 AM							●
4:00 AM					⊕		
5:00 AM						⊕	
6:00 AM	●	●	●	●	●		
7:00 AM	☀	☀	☀	☀	☀	●	
8:00 AM		C	C				●
9:00 AM				C	C	☀	
10:00 AM	C						☀
11:00 AM	C					C	
NOON						C	C
1:00 PM							
2:00 PM		N					
3:00 PM						E	TV
4:00 PM							TV
5:00 PM		N	E				TV
6:00 PM							

KEY

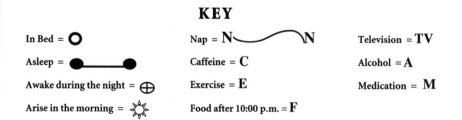

In Bed = ○
Asleep = ●——●
Awake during the night = ⊕
Arise in the morning = ☀

Nap = N⌇N
Caffeine = C
Exercise = E
Food after 10:00 p.m. = F

Television = TV
Alcohol = A
Medication = M

Sleep Log

TIME	SUN–MON	MON–TUES	TUES–WED	WED–THURS	THURS–FRI	FRI–SAT	SAT–SUN
6:00 PM							
7:00 PM							
8:00 PM							
9:00 PM							
10:00 PM							
11:00 PM							
MIDNIGHT							
1:00 AM							
2:00 AM							
3:00 AM							
4:00 AM							
5:00 AM							
6:00 AM							
7:00 AM							
8:00 AM							
9:00 AM							
10:00 AM							
11:00 AM							
NOON							
1:00 PM							
2:00 PM							
3:00 PM							
4:00 PM							
5:00 PM							
6:00 PM							

	MONDAY	TUESDAY	WEDNESDAY	THURSDAY	FRIDAY	SATURDAY	SUNDAY
How did you feel when you woke up? *							
How did you feel during the day?*							
Were you more alert in the morning or evening?							

*Tired------------OK---------Refreshed
   1   2   3   4   5   6   7   8   9   10

APPENDIX E

Lesson from a New Health Professional:

How to Incorporate Habits of Health into
Your Life and Practice

As a cardiologist and New Health Professional, I believe the greatest good I can offer is to help people create health in their lives so they can live to the fullest, unencumbered by disease and medication. Clearly, this is a different perspective than reacting to diseased arteries with CABG surgery, PCI, or the myriad medications we routinely recommend for our patients.

We can and must move beyond fixing and reacting to disease by teaching and practicing Habits of Health so we can free ourselves and our patients from so many of the diseases that afflict us. Our patients and many of us as health care professionals are unhealthy due to overweight, obesity, poor nutrition, lack of exercise, lack of sleep, and enormous stress.

Dr. A's Habits of Health is an invaluable resource, a guide to optimal health that can benefit our profession and our patients. All the technology and medication in the world will never be able to help people create health in their lives. Like the lifeguard who can save a person who is drowning but does not then teach that individual how to swim, we must now move into the Third Era of Medicine, beyond the medications and technology, beyond the fixing and reacting to disease, and bring a paradigm shift into our lives and our practice that will empower us to learn and teach Habits of Health so we can give our patients a prescription for life and health. This is, after all, what our patients want.

As allopathic-trained physicians we focus primarily on disease states, their clinical manifestations, diagnostic and therapeutic tests, procedures, medications, and surgery. We generally don't talk with our patients about their overall health (physical, emotional, mental, and spiritual), much less ask them about the various stressors in their lives, their work, or home environment. We have been trained to be "body mechanics," dealing with the parts of the body that we're called upon to address.

Our technology and medications have a powerful role to play for those who are sick (acutely ill or injured). But we can also be healers. Millions of Americans are in a non-sick state. They don't require medical intervention in the classic sense, but they are often very unhealthy, waiting for the other shoe to drop. We can help both our sick and non-sick patients attain optimal health by teaching them to learn, understand, and facilitate their own body's enormous potential to repair, heal, grow, and create health.

We must invite our patients to embark on a journey alongside us, a journey predicated upon learning that health is more than the absence of disease; health is the ultimate expression of our body's innate capacity to regenerate, heal, create and grow. Our work must be about empowering our patients to live healthy lives so they can thrive and share this creation of health with those they love and care for.

Many of us believe that health is really a mirage, or only the absence of disease. Even if we dare to recognize that optimal health is real and attainable, we will not embark on a journey without a clear path to follow. That path is laid out in *Dr. A's Habits of Health.*